D0056908

1,001 PEARLS OF RUNNERS' WISDOM

Advice and Inspiration for the Open Road

EDITED AND INTRODUCED BY

BILL KATOVSKY

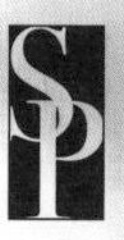

Skyhorse Publishing

"Rejoice, we conquer!"

—from Robert Browning's 1879
poem Pheidippides

Skyhorse Publishing books may be purchased in bulk at special discounts for sales promotion, corporate gifts, fund-raising, or educational purposes. Special editions can also be created to specifications. For details, contact the Special Sales Department, Skyhorse Publishing, 307 West 36th Street, 11th Floor, New York, NY 10018 or info@skyhorsepublishing.com.

Skyhorse® and Skyhorse Publishing® are registered trademarks of Skyhorse Publishing, Inc.®, a Delaware corporation.

www.skyhorsepublishing.com

10 9 8 7 6 5 4 3 2 1

Library of Congress Cataloging-in-Publication Data is available on file.

ISBN: 978-1-61608-712-8

Printed in China

Table of Contents

INTRODUCTION

Before I began the heavy-lifting task of compiling this new collection of quotes about running, I was hard-pressed to even cite a single one by memory. As a middle-aged recreational runner of the "Just Do It" generation, I have certainly come across many of these quotes in running magazines or online. Perhaps my forgetfulness was related to a chronic inability to recall songs or memorize short poems. In fact, the only poem I'm able to recall verbatim contains just 16 words. "The Red Wheelbarrow" by William Carlos Williams goes like this: "So much depends/ upon/ a red wheel/ barrow/ glazed with rain/ water/ beside the white/ chickens." (I had to write an essay on this poem in 11th grade Honors English.)

What that short poem taught me, just like any memorable quote or song lyric can effectively do, is how the right combination of words, even if it's only a short phrase, can make one look at the world differently—to see what is not always readily visible, to peel back the curtain just a tad, and say to oneself, "Hmm, I never thought of that before."

And it's not just words that have that effect on one's powers of perception. Smell is another. I like running after it rains. Where I live in Northern California, the hillside is lined with eucalyptus trees whose leaves give off this amazingly fragrant menthol scent. I often keep my eyes half-shut as I let the bracing aroma waft into my lungs. The olfactory experience reinvigorates my entire being, making the run even more soul-cleansing enjoyable. And because I run without ear buds channeling digitized music inside my skull, Mother Nature is my private concertmaster, soothing me with a symphony of delightful sounds: wind whistling through the pine trees, water happily singing over rocks in the creeks, birds greeting each other in their own avian tongues.

We depend upon our five senses to guide us through life. They are our reliable navigators. But it's usually sight that gets top billing. And nothing is more potent than words that we read on the printed page, computer screen, or tablet.

Words can trick and bamboozle, lure us into rote daily apathy, or stir us into insight and action. When someone says, "Have a nice day," do you really remember what was said an hour later? But what if a runner came up to you in the park or at a race wearing a T-shirt with just a few words printed on the front that said, "We are all an experiment of one"?

I'd wager that this famous George Sheehan quote would ricochet inside your head for a good long while, as you attempted to apply its meaning to your own life and personal commitment to running.

And that's the real hope of this book—to help you look at the multi-faceted world of running through a new and freshly altered filter. The 1,001 Pearls of Runners' Wisdom covers a wide swath of topics, including training, coaching, marathons, diet, and even the latest game-changing trend known as natural running, as well as one inspired by Christopher McDougall's national bestseller, Born to Run. Moreover, this whopping-big collection has another grand purpose: to provide you with a seemingly endless supply of motivational training and racing fodder. This will come in handy if or when the healthy impulse to "Just Do It!" is temporarily sidelined by its black-sheep, La-Z-Boy brother, "Just Screw It!"

By allowing this reference book to become your own workout companion, you will have a reliable ally always at the ready. These quotes have been culled from numerous sources: Olympic champions, coaches, running legends, literature, Hollywood, bloggers, and more.

With 1,001 Pearls of Runners' Wisdom, you can thumb through it at your leisure or when you need to give yourself a quick pep talk like on the eve of an important race. Maybe even record a dozen or so sayings and store them in your iPod. Feel free to experiment, like Dr. Sheehan recommended.

The best way to use this book is by directly going to the chapter that best matches your mood or inclination. While 1,001 Pearls of Runners' Wisdom is organized thematically, with each chapter standing on its own two legs, often a quote resisted being easily categorized. For example, take this quote by retired German long-distance running great Uta Pippig who was the first woman to win the Boston Marathon three consecutive times: "I have the mentality that I can train like a man, and it helps me a lot." Does her statement belong in the Marathon, Training, or Women's Only chapter? After some deliberation, I slotted it in Training. But you will find additional Pippig quotes in other chapters, just as is the case with a number of other quotable runners like Frank Shorter and Bill Rodgers.

Running has such a rich, colorful, and storied heritage that this book easily could have been twice the size. But then, that would have made it too cumbersome to leaf through. And since many people like to read collections of this kind not always sequentially, but often perusing the last chapter first, the final chapter is called Miscellany, and it's just that—a random, eclectic, and invigorating assortment of quotes that should give one a virtual runner's high.

Finally, do I have a personal favorite quote? Hmm, that's a tough call. There are so many great, memorable sayings in this book, including those voiced by Olympic, long-distance champions (Emil Zatopek and Sebastian Coe), legendary coaches (Bill Bowerman and Percy Cerutty), and female running-trailblazers (Kathy Switzer and Joan Benoit Samuelson). But, if forced to choose just one, it would probably belong to the late Walt Stack, who said, "Start slowly and taper off." It's also the long-time, official motto of the Dolphin South End Runners, the oldest and largest running club in San Francisco, which was founded by Stack in 1966.

For 27 years, from 1966–1993, Stack, a retired, merchant seaman, would begin almost every day in San Francisco the same way: bicycle six miles from his home to the Golden Gate Bridge, strip to his shorts, run bare-chested across the bridge to Sausalito and back, and follow that jaunt with a 30 minute swim in the cold, San Francisco Bay. He followed this routine year round—cold, heat, fog, rain, wind—and always shirtless. When he founded the Dolphin South End Runners Club, its symbol was a turtle and the motto, "Start Off Slow and Taper Off."

A guy who only started running when he turned 58, Walt ran in over 70 marathons (with times ranging from 3:30 to 4:00), eight 50-milers, and a 100-miler. "There was a time," he told one running magazine reporter during a 17-mile workout, that "When I figured I'd like to run around the world in terms of miles, but I passed that 24,000-mile mark some years back, so that's nothing now. I'd just like to keep in fair shape and do it as long as I can without strain."

Stack's Ironman-like exploits (he did the Hawaii Ironman triathlon once, in February 1982, taking 26 hours to complete it) earned him guest appearances on "The Tonight Show With Johnny Carson," an endorsement of a new $69 waterproof watch sold in the Sharper Image catalog, and the honor of being featured in Nike's first "Just Do It" television commercial.

In 1983, I met Walt in Kona while I was covering the Hawaii Ironman for a magazine I founded called Tri-Athlete. *Walt wasn't competing that year. Incidentally, the Ironman officials had instituted the "Walt Stack" rule that stipulated a 17-hour mandatory deadline for all racers. He was weathered-looking but very much in admirable shape, his tanned muscular chest covered with faded tattoos of birds, horses, and women in bathing suits. I remember his language being colorful, salty and ribald. He was old-school, politically incorrect, and outspoken.*

Six months earlier, Stack had celebrated his 75th birthday in splendid, ceremonial style. San Francisco Mayor Dianne Feinstein had declared it "Walt Stack Day" and 3,000 runners crossed the 1.1-mile long Golden Gate Bridge with him. They all went at Walt's speed—a slow, steady, foot-shuffling jog. No one was in a hurry that day.

Walt continued the same daily workout regimen for another decade. Eventually, old age caught up with him and he was forced to give up biking, running, and swimming. He had earned the right to taper. He died at the age of 87 in a nursing home.

Walt's carpe diem lifestyle embodied a simple universal

truth: The finish line is the same for all runners. How we get there and what we do along the way are what matters most. The journey defines us.

—Bill Katovsky,

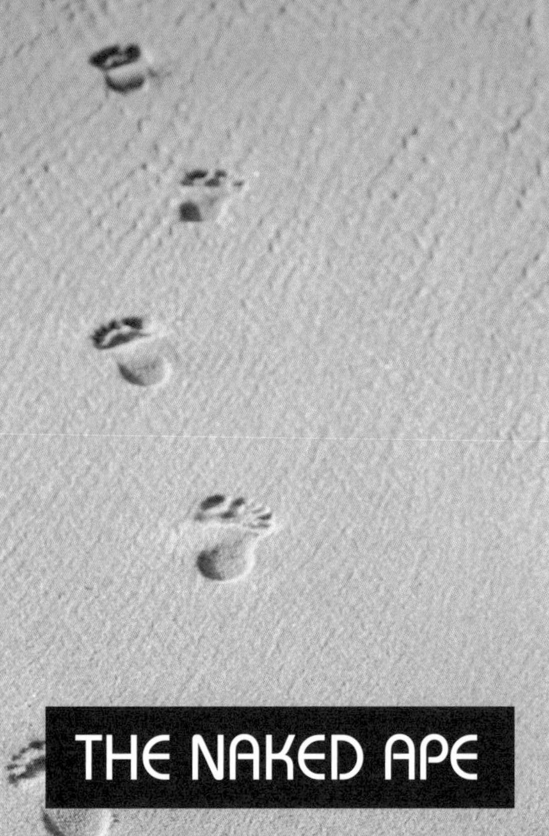

THE NAKED APE

The next time you come back from a long run, dripping with sweat, sunburned, and calves aching from exertion, you should stop complaining and instead show some appreciation for evolution since it ensured you have the right kind of body to be an endurance athlete. Ever since early man first branched off from his ape-like lineage and became a bipedal hominid on the move, natural selection has steered the human genome towards enhanced efficiency when it comes to terrestrial locomotion.

By comparison, our closest, living, primate cousin, the chimpanzee (we share 98 percent of the same genes) is a close-to-home fellow, seldom venturing far in search of food or suitable mate. Chimps use their feet primarily for grasping and climbing, and their simian anatomy would not make it easy for them to walk or run very far. Their big toes are long, and not anatomically designed for upright balance and running. They have very few tendons in their lower legs that can act like spring-coiled shock absorbers when their feet hit the ground during the act of running. And because their bodies are covered with thick hair that impedes sweating and evaporation, they'd overheat from sustained physical exertion. In other words, chimps aren't born to become endurance runners. Only humans are.

The Naked Ape

Distance running was the way we survived and thrived and spread across the planet. You ran to eat and to avoid being eaten; you ran to find a mate and impress her, and with her you ran off to start a new life together. You had to love running, or you wouldn't live to love anything else. [Running] is really an encoded ancestral necessity.

—Christopher McDougall, author of *Born to Run: A Hidden Tribe, Superathletes, and the Greatest Race the World Has Never Seen*

There is nothing quite so gentle, deep, and irrational as our running—and nothing quite so savage, and so wild.

—Bernd Heinrich, Ph.D., author of *Why We Run: A Natural History*

We are inherently more like wolves than lapdogs, because the communal chase is part of our biological makeup.

—Bernd Heinrich

If walking upright first set early human ancestors apart from their ape cousins, it may have been their eventual ability to run long distances with a springing step over the African savanna that influenced the transition to today's human body form.

—John Noble Wilford, *New York Times* science writer

Running is the most elemental sport there is. We are genetically programmed to do it. One might even say we are the free-ranging, curious, restless creatures that we are because of running.

—John Jerome, prolific fitness and travel author

There are 193 species of monkeys and apes, 192 of them are covered with hair. The exception is a naked ape self-named *Homo sapiens.*

—Desmond Morris, best-selling British author of *The Naked Ape* and *The Human Zoo*

The Naked Ape

I run because I am an animal. I run because it is part of my genetic wiring. I run because millions of years of evolution have left me programmed to run. And, finally, I run because there's no better way to see the sun rise and set.

—Amby Burfoot

Endurance? You've only got to get out there and do it. Face up to it: Man was meant to run.

—Percy Cerutty, legendary Australian running coach

I put it in historical perspective. This is our heritage; our evolutionary gift, dating back to our days as hunters and gatherers.

—Stu Mittleman, winner of the 1,000-Mile World Championship (11 days, 20 hours, 36 minutes) in 1986

Being fit isn't about being able to lift a steel bar or finish an Ironman. It's about rediscovering our biological nature and releasing the wild human animal inside.

—Erwan Le Corre, quoted in Christopher McDougall's profile of the MovNat founder in *Men's Health*

You never see your dog running nonstop around and around in a circle for an hour. If he did, you'd think there was something wrong with him. Instead, he'll chase something, roll around, sprint, rest, mix things up. Animal play has a purpose, and it's not hard to surmise that human play should as well.

—Erwan Le Corre

Running is like going to a spring: Each of us drinks our fill, and new runners come, pushing aside those in front.

—Michael Sandrock, running journalist and author

There is no substitute for learning to live in our bodies. All the tests and all the machines in the world will fail if we do not first become good animals.

—George Sheehan, M.D.

The freedom of cross-country is so primitive. It's woman vs. nature.

—Lynn Jennings, one of the best female American distance runners of all time

Our ability to move for long distances at sub-maximal speeds is a gift to our species, like language.

—Stu Mittleman

If you have very long toes, the moment of force acting on the foot's metatarsal phalangeal joint becomes problematic when running. [Our hominid ancestor *Australopithecus*] Lucy could have walked just fine with her long toes. But if she wanted to run a marathon, or even a half-marathon, she'd have had trouble.

—Daniel Lieberman, Professor of Human Evolutionary Biology at Harvard University, aka "The Barefoot Professor"

Running was mankind's first fine art, our original act of inspired creation. Way before we were scratching pictures on caves or beating rhythms on hollow trees, we were perfecting the art of combining our breath and mind and muscles into fluid self-propulsion over wild terrain.

—Christopher McDougall

I feel like trail running is so healthy. It's like going to the farmers' market for your lungs. You just feel so healthy coming out of the woods versus coming off the roads. I love the track, but I crave trails. I get hungry, thirsty, itchy for the woods . . . the moss, the dampness.

—Joan Nesbit Mabe, 1995 US Cross-Country National Champion and former Olympian

Just move your legs. Because if you don't think you were born to run, you're not only denying history; you're denying who you are.

—Dr. Dennis Bramble, University of Utah biologist, quoted in *Born to Run*

The Naked Ape

Name any other athletic endeavor where sixty-four-year-olds are competing with nineteen-year-olds. Swimming? Boxing? Not even close. There's something really weird about us humans: We're not only really good at endurance running; we're really good at it for a remarkably long time.

—Dr. Dennis Bramble

Millions of years of genetic mutation and adaptation have produced a singular animal whose body, mind, and spirit are primed to sprint as if life depended on it. That animal is you. So why are you just standing there?

—Richard Conniff, *Men's Health* contributing writer

Versatility was the key to survival, because early humans had to be ready for anything at any time. If your daily life is hunting and being hunted, at a moment's notice you might have to sprint, jog, throw a spear, scramble up a tree, hunker down, and dig. The specialization we enjoy today, be it as a marathoner or a tennis player — even a triathlete — is a luxury of modern society. It doesn't have great survival value for *Homo sapiens* in the wild.

—E. Paul Zehr, Ph.D, author of *Becoming Batman: The Possibility of a Superhero* as quoted in Christopher McDougall's profile of Erwan Le Corre in Men's Health

Remember guys, there's more to moving naturally than just running.

—Erwan Le Corre

It has been said that the love of the chase is an inherent delight in man—a relic of an instinctive passion.

—Charles Darwin

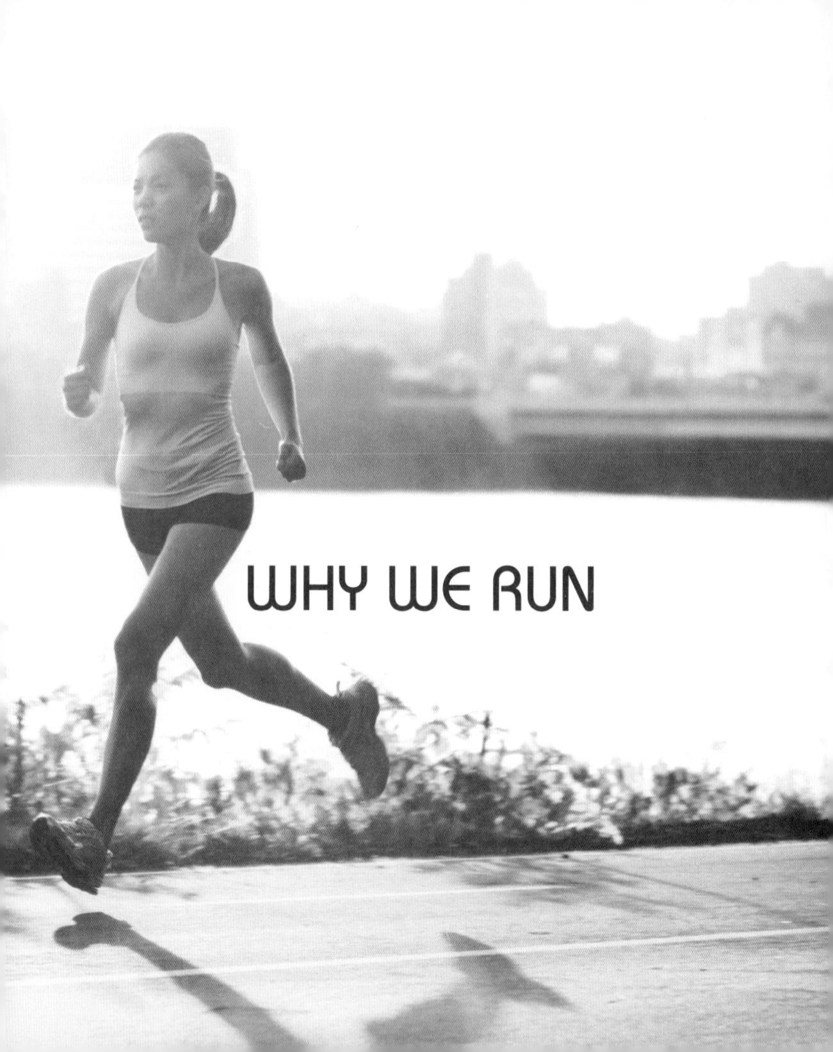

WHY WE RUN

Let's jump right in. No time to waste or dilly-dally. If you are thumbing through this book, it's almost certain that you are already a runner. You don't need advice on how to get started. You already made that commitment. What you do want to read is why others run. What motivates them to wake up before dawn and head outside with a Petzl headlamp guiding their foot-strikes in the inky dark? Or what makes the great runners tick?

The seventeenth century, French philosopher Rene Descartes wrote "Cogito, ergo sum." *Translated in English, it is, "I think, therefore I am." For runners, that phrase can be revised to, "I run, therefore I am."*

Have you ever felt worse after a run?

—George Sheehan, M.D., best-selling author

Newsman: Sir, why are you running?
1st Reporter: Why are you running?
2nd Reporter: Are you doing this for world peace?
3rd Reporter: Are you doing this for women's rights?
Newsman: Or for the environment?
Reporter: Or for animals?
3rd Reporter: Or for nuclear arms?
2nd Reporter: Why are you doing this?
Forrest Gump: I just felt like running.

—from the movie *Forrest Gump*

Being a runner means you are now 'free' to win and lose and live life to its fullest.

—Bill Rodgers, four-time winner of
Boston and New York City Marathons

When I'm running I don't have to talk to anybody and don't have to listen to anybody. This is a part of my day I can't do without.

—Haruki Murakami, novelist and author of *What I Talk About When I Talk About Running*

Running defines me. It is a euphoric feeling I look forward to every day. It keeps me connected to life. And every November I get to witness the outpouring of compassion and spirit that this city gives to thousands of runners who tackle our marathon.

—Allan Steinfield, former race director of New York City Marathon

Running made me feel like a bird let out of a cage, I loved it that much.

—Priscilla Welch, started running at age 35 and winner of New York City Marathon

As a boy, running was always pure joy for me. When I ran I would just let my mind wander and drift. But I would concentrate, too. I would imagine I could fly: *Run harder,* I would tell myself. *I know I can make a life of my own away from this farm.*

—Haile Gebrselassie, two-time Olympic gold medalist in the 10,000 meters and former world record holder for the marathon

Running is not a crime. Running is a revolution. Don't believe the propaganda or the rumors from the non-running status quo. There is no proof of a Nixon-appointed task force monitoring the effects of the runner's high. Running is not addictive. By now you know, running is a way of life.

—from 1977 issue of *Oregon Runner* magazine

For the most part, we exist in a numb, dead society. I'm doing my best to be alive and running in the mountains is the best way I've found to do that. And because I love the effortlessness that sometimes occurs while cruising down a cushy pine-needle singletrack or even while grinding up a switchback above tree line. I love how I can run up and into a mountain cirque or over a pass and be completely dwarfed and humbled by the sheer immensity and grandiosity of the landscape and I love flying down the other side with the breeze in my hair and the gravel in my shoes and the burning in my quads and the branches in my face and then when I'm finally all worn out there's nothing like peeling my shoes off and just sitting. Just being at rest. Running sharpens the focus on life and intensifies the emotions. Is there any better reason to do anything?

—Anton Krupicka, two-time winner of Leadville 100

I was born to be a runner. I simply love to run.

—Mary Decker-Slaney, holder of 36 U.S. middle-distance records

Running has made being depressed impossible. If I'm going through something emotional and just go outside for a run, you can rest assured I'll come back with clarity.

—Alanis Morissette, singer and actress

I run for the variety it puts into my life. I'm a teacher, writer, scholar and administrator; my work is intellectual and sedentary. Running is physical and mobile. Work is complicated — reports, reviews, theories, controversies, demands, budgets. Running is simple. A loose shoe on a muddy day is your worst problem. Work is done for others: students, readers, presidents, ministers. Running is for me. Work is a duty, a constraint. Running is free.

—Roger Robinson, New Zealand writer, English professor, and competitive runner for over 50 years

I always loved running... it was something you could do by yourself, and under your own power. You could go in any direction, fast or slow as you wanted, fighting the wind if you felt like it, seeking out new sights just on the strength of your feet and the courage of your lungs.

—Jesse Owens, winner of four gold medals at the 1936 Berlin Olympics

When I run the roads, I am a saint. For that hour, I am an Assisi wearing the least and meanest of clothes. I am Gandhi, the young London law student, trotting 10 or 12 miles a day and then going to a cheap restaurant to eat his fill of bread. I am Thoreau, the solitary seeking union with the world around him.

—George Sheehan, M.D.

If Frank Shorter inspired the first running boom, Oprah inspired the second, by running the Marine Corps Marathon. And it was a much bigger boom. This was not a spindly 24-year-old Yalie gliding through Old World Munich. If Oprah could run a marathon, shame on anyone who couldn't.

—Edward McClelland, author and journalist

A lot of people say they love running because of how they feel afterward. Not me. Well, I love that, too, but it's also so much fun while I'm out there."

—Dick Beardsley, 1981 London Marathon champion and inducted into the National Distance Running Hall of Fame

For me, running is a lifestyle and an art. I'm more interested in the magic of it than the mechanics.

—Lorraine Moller, four-time New Zealand Olympian

I run because it's how I keep the black dog of depression from nipping at my heels.

—Bill Katovsky, two-time Hawaii Ironman finisher, author, and editor of *1,001 Pearls of Running Wisdom*

Jogging is very beneficial. It's good for your legs and your feet. It's also very good for the ground. It makes it feel needed.

—Charles Schulz, *Peanuts*

This is what really matters: running. This is where I know where I am.

—Steve Jones, former world record holder in the marathon, and winner at the London, Chicago (twice), and New York City Marathons

I run in order to acquire a void. The thoughts that occur to me while I'm running are like clouds in the sky. Clouds of all different sizes. They come and they go, while the sky remains the same sky as always.

—Haruki Murakami

Running is ultimately a personal experience. It is a revival of the spirit, a private oasis for the thirsty mind. Yet, its healing power only increases in the presence of others. Run together and the oasis grows cooler and more satisfying.

—Amby Burfoot, author, former editor-at-large at *Runner's World,* and winner of the 1968 Boston Marathon

Out on the roads there is fitness and self-discovery and the persons we were destined to be.

—George Sheehan, M.D.

It's how I get a front-row seat to the calming, enjoyable spectacle of experiencing endorphins as they do their magical tap-dance inside my brain.

—Bill Katovsky

Every day, I stop halfway through my run for five minutes, look around, and enjoy the surroundings. I'm reminded of why I do this and why I love it so much.

—Anita Ortiz, 45, mother of four, won the 2008 Western States 100

The desire to run comes from deep within us— from the unconscious, the instinctive, the intuitive.

—George Sheehan, M.D.

The number of miles I have run since I was a toddler would have taken me around the world several times, and I still cannot define precisely my joy in running. There is no sacrifice in it. I lead what I regard a normal life. In my case, I thoroughly enjoy running 100-odd miles a week. If I didn't I wouldn't do it. Who can define happiness? To some, happiness is a warm puppy or a glass of cold beer. To me, happiness is running in the hills with my mates around me.

—Ron Clarke, Australian distance runner and first man to break the 28-minute barrier in the 10,000 meters (27:39.4)

What am I doing—nobody cares. It's just personal satisfaction.

—Kenny Moore, journalist and American fourth-place finisher in the 1972 Olympic Marathon

When we run, we are already so exposed, often nearly naked in our shorts and T-shirts, huffing and puffing, purified by the effort. Briefly removed from the defenses and secrets we maintain in so much of our lives, we feel less need to hide our private thoughts, loves, fears, and stresses. We share.

—Amby Burfoot

If I don't run, I'll get fat again.

—Dave Low, winner of Hawaii's Fittest CEO competition, had lost 75 pounds

I can't imagine living and not running.

—Paula Radcliffe, three-time winner of the London Marathon and two-time New York Marathon champion

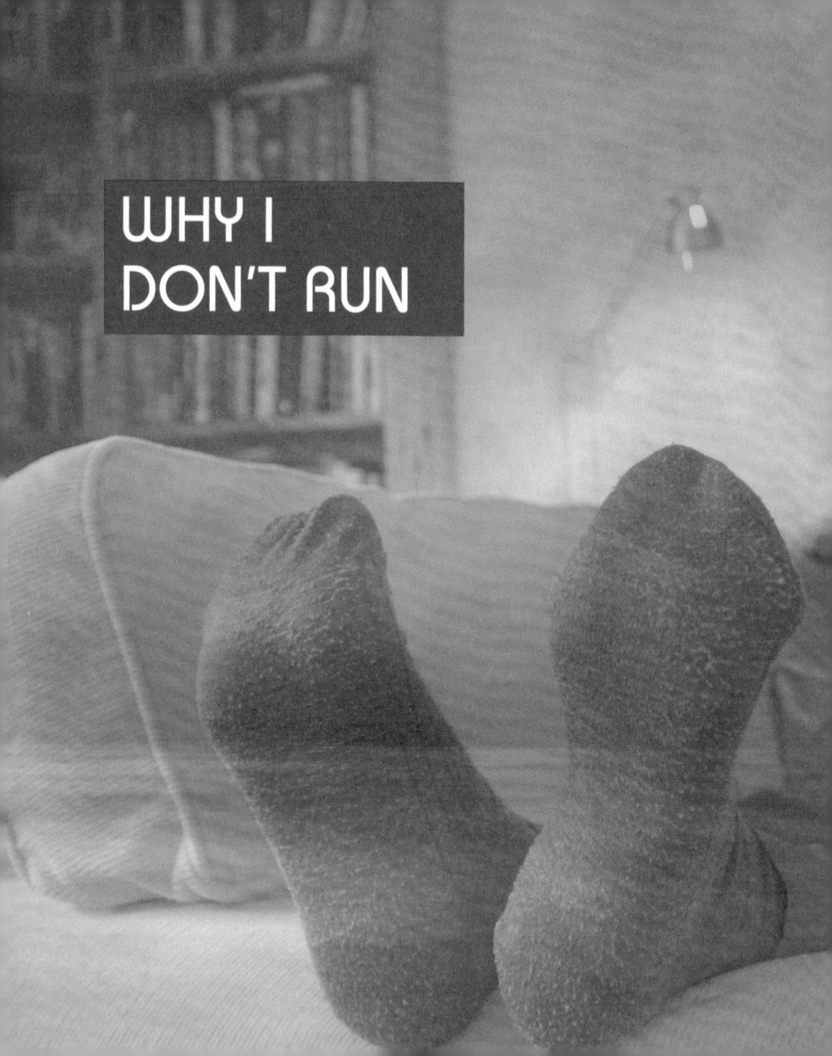
WHY I
DON'T RUN

Then there are the naysayers and cynics, the self-satisfied and smug couch potatoes who sneer at the foreign concepts of sweat and exercise. But these anti-runners are only hiding behind the shields of their own insecurities. That explains why they criticize and scoff. And if a marathon runner happens to have a fatal heart attack during a race, the media is notoriously complicit in raising the alarm that running can be deadly. These detractors and doubters are then quick to cite that unfortunate tragedy as a way to shore up their own false senses of sedentary superiority.

Then why even include their quotes in this collection of wise, wonderful, and witty running quotes? Certainly, these insalubrious viewpoints are a case of swine before pearls. But their presence can serve a cathartic purpose, as you say to yourself, "I'm not like them. I like running!" To be fair, however, many of these quotes are the product of a comic imagination. Think of them as one-liners. It's okay to suppress a chuckle or LOL.

Health nuts are going to feel stupid someday, lying in hospitals dying of nothing.

—Redd Foxx, comic

The pleasure of jogging and running is rather like that of wearing a fur coat in Texas in August: the true joy comes in being able to take the damn thing off.

—Joseph Epstein, essayist

I don't jog. If I die I want to be sick.

—Abe Lemons, college basketball coach

It's unnatural for people to run around the city streets unless they are thieves or victims. It makes people nervous to see someone running. I know that when I see someone running on my street, my instincts tell me to let the dog go after him.

—Mike Royko, Chicago newsman

I don't generally like running. I believe in training by rising gently up and down from the bench.

—Satchel Paige, baseball pitcher

It must be spring; the saps are running.

—old saying, in reference to the Boston Marathon

I don't think jogging is healthy, especially morning jogging. If morning joggers knew how tempting they looked to morning motorists, they would stay home and do sit-ups.

—Rita Rudner, comic

I believe that the Good Lord gave us a finite number of heartbeats and I'm damned if I'm going to use up mine running up and down a street.

—Neil Armstrong, astronaut

Dick Cheney said he was running again. He said his health was fine. "I've got a doctor with me twenty-four hours a day." Yeah, that's always the sign of a man in good health, isn't it?

—David Letterman, TV talk-show host

The first time I see a jogger smiling, I'll consider it.

—Joan Rivers, ageless comic

Have you ever noticed? Anyone going slower than you is an idiot, and anyone going faster than you is a maniac?

—George Carlin, comic

The trouble with jogging is that the ice falls out of your glass.

—Martin Mull, comic

My doctor recently told me that jogging could add years to my life. I think he was right. I feel ten years older already.

—Milton Berle, comic

"Ruin Your Knees for Charity"

—sign on Springfield Marathon starting-line banner in *The Simpsons*

The only reason I would take up jogging is so that I could hear heavy breathing again.

—Erma Bombeck, newspaper columnist

Why I Don't Run

When it comes to sports I am not particularly interested. Generally speaking, I look upon them as dangerous and tiring activities performed by people with whom I share nothing except the right to trial by jury.

—Fran Lebowitz, humorist and professional procrastinator

Whenever I get the urge to exercise, I lie down until the feeling passes away.

—Robert M. Hutchins, former President of the University of Chicago.

I am sick of joggers and I am sick of runners. I don't care if all the people in the U.S. are running or planning to run or wishing they could run. All I ask is, don't write articles about running and ask me to read them.

—Frank Deford, *Sports Illustrated* writer, in 1978

I have never taken any exercise, except for sleeping and resting, and I never intend to take any. Exercise is loathsome.

—Mark Twain, author and humorist

Oh yes, I will work out today. I will work out a way to avoid running for a stupid cause.

—Stanley, from *The Office*

Exercise is a modern superstition invented by people who ate too much, and had nothing to think about. Athletics don't make anybody either long-lived or useful.

—George Santayana, philosopher

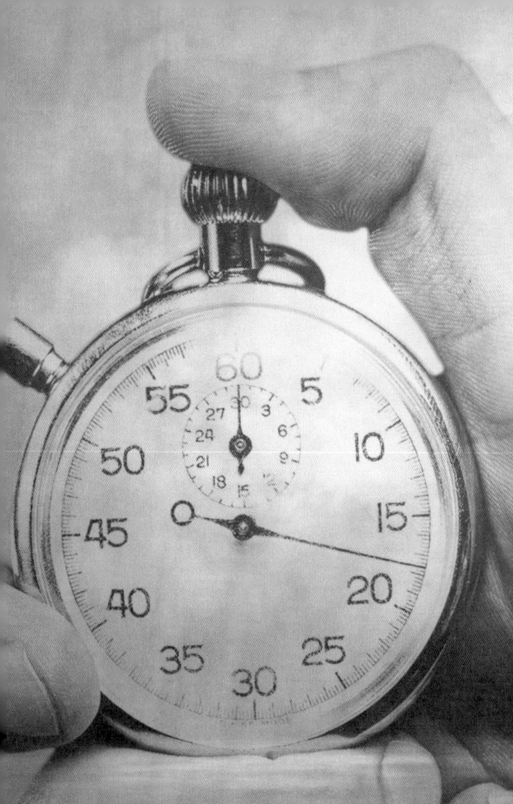

PRESS START

"A journey of a thousand miles begins with a single step." You have probably read or heard that quotation before. It comes from the Chinese philosopher Lao Tzu who lived over 2,500 years ago. That makes it the oldest quote in this collection, and also one of the most important sayings for the beginning runner.

We all remember when we decided to become runners for the very first time, and what it felt like in the beginning—the awkwardness, unfamiliarity, and the leg tiredness that accompanied the uncertainty of making it through those early, embryonic miles. But as your training, conditioning, and self-confidence steadily improved, you began to create new goals and challenges to test your potential. Running soon became the most natural thing in the world.

Or maybe you once were a runner in your youth but gave up the sport when job or family intervened, and you haven't run in years. Your body went soft and spherical. Weight accumulated in the wrong places. Now you want to shed that excess poundage and start running again, but desire and doing live two very different lives. The latter might require coaxing and encouragement. If so, allow the quotes in this chapter to offer assistance and help you conquer those first thousand miles. The next thousand miles will be much easier.

Press Start

At age forty-three, when I found myself standing in my garage in a new pair of running shoes, I knew that it was my moment of truth . . . Behind me lay forty years of bad decisions and broken promises.

—John Bingham, author of *The Courage to Start*

When I first started running, I was so embarrassed I'd walk when cars passed me. I'd pretend I was looking at the flowers.

—Joan Benoit-Samuelson, won the first-ever women's marathon at the 1984 Los Angeles Olympics

That day, for no particular reason, I decided to go for a little run. So, I ran to the end of the road, and when I got there, I thought maybe I'd run to the end of town. And when I got there, I thought maybe I'd just run across Greenbow County. And I figured since I run this far, maybe I'd just run across the great state of Alabama. And that's what I did. I ran clear across Alabama. For no particular reason, I just kept on going. I ran clear to the ocean. And when I got there, I figured since I'd gone this far, I might as well turn around, just keep on going. When I got to another ocean, I figured since I've gone this far, I might as well just turn back, keep right on going. When I got tired, I slept. When I got hungry, I ate. When I had to go, you know, I went. My mama always said you got to put the past behind you before you can move on. And I think that's what my running was all about. I had run for three years, two months, 14 days, and 16 hours.

—Forrest Gump, from the movie *Forrest Gump*

I protested that I was weak and not fit to run, but the coach sent me for a physical examination and the doctor said that I was perfectly well. So I had to run, and when I got started I felt I wanted to win. But I only came in second. That was the way it started.

—Emil Zatopek, Czech running legend and winner of three gold medals at the 1952 Helsinki Olympics (5,000 meters, 10,000 meters, marathon)

I began running on an everyday basis after I became a writer. As being a writer requires sitting at a desk for hours a day, without getting some exercise you'd quickly get out of shape and gain weight, I figured. That was 22 years ago. I also took it as a chance to quit smoking. You see, I became rapidly healthier since the time I became a writer. You may call it rather a rare case. But because of that, I weigh now just as much as I weighed back then.

—Haruki Murakami

I'm afraid the reason so many new runners quit is because they never get past the point of feeling like they have to run.

—John Bingham

I was embarrassed that I was so small. I wanted to build up my body. My husband helped me go to the gym where he was a member, and I began to run. I had strange looks. Someone told me I should be home in the kitchen. But I had one mentor, and he encouraged me to enter a 100-mile/24-hour indoors race, in the gym. Yes, hundreds of laps. The first year I stopped at 86 miles. I cried.

—Miki Gorman, two-time winner of Boston and New York City Marathons

It's very hard in the beginning to understand that the whole idea is not to beat the other runners. Eventually you learn that the competition is against the little voice inside you that wants to quit.

—George Sheehan, M.D.

Starting is scary. It is for everyone. I never allowed my eyes to meet those of other runners, because I was afraid of seeming like an impostor.

—John Bingham

Generally slow running is considered jogging, but I think you're better off considering yourself a runner from the start.

—Marc Bloom, *The Runner's Bible*

All runners, at one time or another, are beginners.

—from *New York Road Runner's Club Complete Book of Running*

If you want to become the best runner you can be, start now. Don't spend the rest of your life wondering if you can do it.

—Priscella Welch

The advice I have for beginners is the same philosophy that I have for runners of all levels of experience and ability—consistency, a sane approach, moderation and making your running an enjoyable, rather than dreaded, part of your life.

—Bill Rodgers

In the beginning you likely say, "I run." With more confidence, you say, "I am a runner."

—Gloria Averbuch, author of health, fitness and running books

My first understanding was that you could not become a distance runner quickly. I began gradually, not doing too much.

—Henry Rono, broke four world records in 81 days: 10,000 meters, 5,000 meters, 3,000 meters steeplechase, and the 3,000 meters

Set a goal and a program for yourself, and everything else will follow. Guaranteed.

—Amby Burfoot

On my first day as a runner, I owned nine motorcycles, two cars, a camper, a garden tractor, a riding lawn mower, and a gas-powered weed whacker. I was never in danger of having to exert myself.

—John Bingham

For the novice runner, I'd say to give yourself at least two months of consistently running several times a week at a conversational pace before deciding whether you want to stick with it. Consistency is the most important aspect of training at this point.

—Frank Shorter, winner of the 1972 Olympic marathon and silver medalist in the 1976 Olympic marathon

I always tell beginning runners: Train your brain first. It's much more important than your heart or legs.

—Amby Burfoot

He was too small for football and he got tired of sitting on the bench all the time.

—Ray Prefontaine, on how his son Steve got interested in running

It was back in 1901, at the age of 21, when I first became interested in distance running. While attending a smoker at the University of Vermont to pep up enthusiasm for a football game, one of the speakers—a Professor Stetson of the German Department—urged all men to try different sports they could be a champion at. At once I wondered what I could be tops at. By a process of elimination, I went out for cross-country.

—Clarence DeMar, winner of seven Boston Marathons

When I went up to Oxford, I wanted to take part in sport. I was too light for rowing, and I wasn't skilled enough for rugby. But I knew I could run.

—Roger Bannister, first person to break the four-minute mile

When I was 12 or 13, the first day I went out, there was a mile cross country race on and they said 'You can't compete, you're too young,' because it was a race with 18-year-olds and like that, and I cried, literally cried, because they wouldn't let me run the race. So they said, 'Okay,' and I beat all these guys who were 18 and over, because I wanted to accept the challenge.

—Eamonn Coghlan, of Ireland, and three-time Olympian and world-champion in the 5,000 meters

It is not so much that I began to run, but that I continued.

—Hal Higdon, prolific author of running books, with over 100 marathon finishes

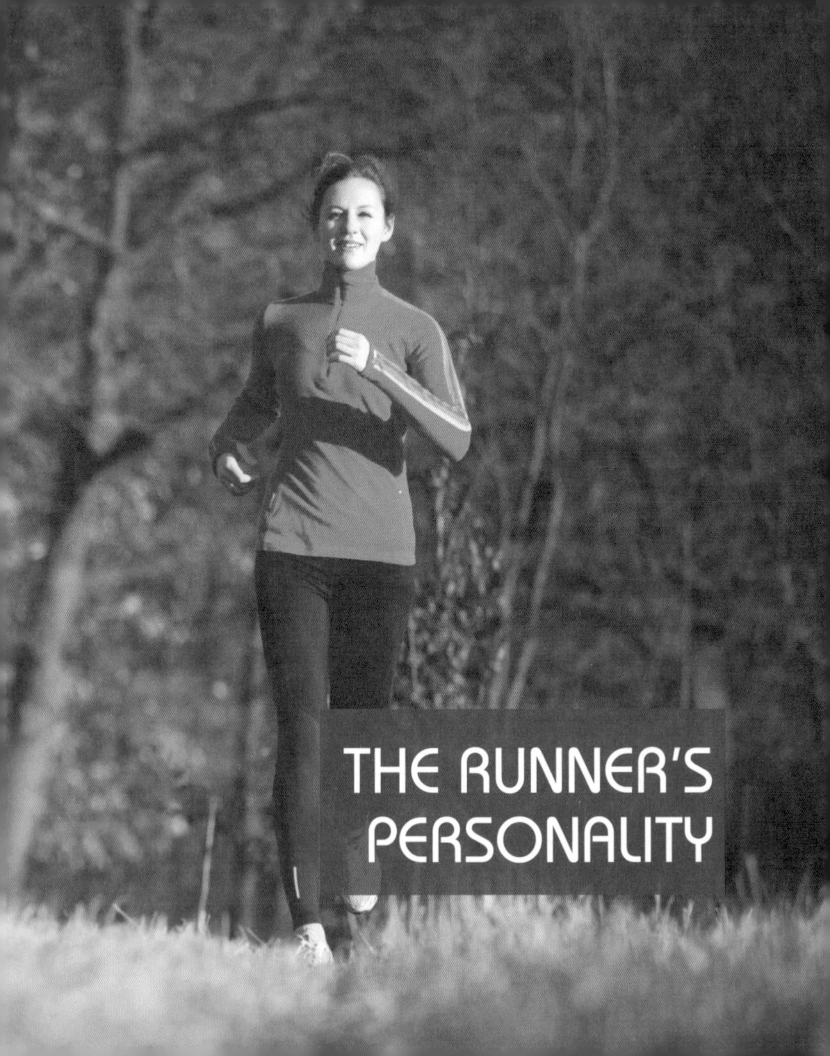

THE RUNNER'S PERSONALITY

Runners are like a moveable Rorschach test in the eyes of non-runners. We're the curious objects of an interpretative guessing game as to what fuels our dedication to running. But to say that all runners are alike or have an addictive, Type-A personality is like saying everyone who lives in Chicago has blonde hair and blue eyes.

No longer is the runner defined by its outdated stereotype—an undernourished gazelle in Nike waffle trainers, high-tube socks and cotton shorts. In the late 1970s, fewer than 30,000 runners completed a marathon in the U.S., which is about 15,000 fewer than the number that raced in the New York City Marathon in 2010. Today's runner is old, young, mom-on-the-go, ex-jock on a mid-life athletic rebound, hard-bodied, pear-shaped, highly competitive, or one who considers "running" 26.2 miles as climbing his or her own Everest, even if takes five or six hours.

What all runners have in common is a deep, atavistic love of forward motion. We're rapt pupils of basic algebra whose sole curriculum revolves around calculating distance, rate, and time. We're constantly traveling from point A to point B, unless we're obsessively committed to running in place on a treadmill, or going in geometric circles around the track.

At big-city runapolooza events, we tentatively find our tiny, personal space amid the collective herd, while waiting anxiously for that exhilarating moment of pure energy release. Although we stand united at the starting line, once the race begins we run alone.

When describing the meaning of existentialism, the poet Delmore Schwartz wrote, "It means that no one else can take a bath for you." It's the same with being a runner. Running means that no one else can do it for you.

Why did I get seriously involved in running? I can't put my finger on one specific thing. I became a runner because it suited my personality. It suited me as an individual. There may be a lot of different reasons, but, somehow, they all came together.

—Bill Rodgers

The human body rather likes routine. So I run out of a dull old daily habit at the stroke of noon with familiar friends on familiar ground. It's a well-established ritual. But today's routine is tomorrow's nostalgia. If the day comes when I can no longer satisfy that old craving, I dare not think how much I shall miss it.

—Roger Robinson

Together, [Bill Rodgers and Frank Shorter] inspired America in its great running boom. And having done that, they seemed tinged by faint embarrassment. Perhaps they just didn't want it to look like they had *ordered* everyone into the streets.

—Kenny Moore

The world is divided into two kinds of people: runners and non-runners.

—Marc Bloom, *The Runner's Bible*

I can't remember what I was doing before running. I guess shopping, sewing, watching TV—gaining nothing.

—Miki Gorman

We may train or peak for a certain race, but running is a lifetime sport.

—Alberto Salazar, three-time winner of the New York City Marathon

Initially, he took pains to hide the fact that he was running at all. Running in public would have been viewed as subversive in a town such as ours—perhaps in any town. Thus he began his running in the privacy of our backyard.

—Andrew Sheehan, writing about his father George Sheehan, M.D. in the early 60s

Somebody once asked me what I would do when I could no longer run. During the 10 minutes of silence that followed, I realized I had never even considered that possible. That was the most depressing question anyone ever asked me!

—Steven Sashen, All-American Master sprinter and developer of Xero Shoes running sandals

The 1960s was a decade both dark with despair and bright with hope, an era when the Boston Marathon attracted only a few hundred starters, most of them capable of breaking three hours. Nineteen fifty-nine was the year I ran my first Boston. We were a scurvy lot, the 150 of us who showed up in Hopkinton, our deeds largely unheralded.

—Hal Higdon

My suspicion is that the effects of running are not extraordinary at all, but quite ordinary. As runners, I think we reach directly back along the endless chain of history.

—James W. Fixx, author of *The Complete Book of Running*

Running is the kind of sport where, once it becomes part of your daily routine, there's very little attrition. That's what sets the running boom apart from other booms.

—Frank Shorter won the marathon at the 1972 Munich Olympics, and was U.S. national 10,000-meters champion four times

They are different personalities, but each wanted to be the best he possibly could be and beat the other guy.

—Amby Burfoot on Bill Rodgers and Frank Shorter

People sometimes sneer at those who run every day, claiming they'll go to any length to live longer. But don't think that's the reason most people run. Most runners run not because they want to live longer, but because they want to live life to the fullest. If you're going to while away the years, it's far better to live them with clear goals and fully alive than in a fog, and I believe running helps you to do that.

—Haruki Murakami

In running, it doesn't matter whether you come in first, in the middle of the pack, or last. You can say, 'I have finished.' There is a lot of satisfaction in that.

—Fred Lebow, founder of New York City Marathon

In the late 1960s and early '70s, those of us who had discovered the rewards of long-distance running were a very obscure minority — unknown to the general population. Sometimes when guys in cars saw us running along the roads in our gym shorts, they'd yell out the window, "What are you running in your underwear for? Hah, hah!" Once, a guy threw a half-full can of beer at me. We didn't let it faze us, though. We were tough!

—Ed Ayres, co-founder of *Running Times*

Running is a thing worth doing not because of the future rewards it bestows, but because of how it feeds our bodies and minds and souls in the present.

—Kevin Nelson, *The Runner's Book of Daily Inspiration*

Running is a fad. Just like breathing is a fad.

—Ben Cheever, author of *Strides: Running Through History With an Unlikely Athlete*

In running (like religion), it's the converts who are likely to exhibit the most zeal. And for that reason, the continuing influx of average beginning runners will always be the lifeblood of this sport.

—Mark Will-Weber, former editor of *Runner's World*

In England, the running club is the hub of your whole social life. It's the hub of your whole damn life.

—Dave Welch

Given the nature of running, certain things will never be altered. That's one of the beauties of our sport. There is no judge; it doesn't matter how you look.

—Bill Rodgers

As runners, we all go through many transitions—transitions that closely mimic the larger changes we experience in a lifetime. First, we try to run faster. Then we try to run harder. Then we learn to accept ourselves and our limitations, and at last, we can appreciate the true joy and meaning of running.

—Amby Burfoot

The Sprinter

The following quotes are from Steven Sashen, 50, an All-American Masters sprinter and founder of Xero Shoes.

Sprinters are born, not made. But sprinting is taught.

Raw speed helps, but it rarely wins.

People who know I'm a sprinter will still say to me, "Hey, let's go for a run." I reply, "I don't run. I sprint.""

Masters sprinters are great fun. We work way too hard for no real payoff, we can't help being way more competitive than we have any reason to be, and we're old enough to know that we're crazy.

The quietest moment in my mind is the space between "Set!" and "BANG!"

Running isn't rocket science. Sprinting comes pretty close.

The reason sprinting isn't more popular than jogging is that anyone can jog.

Saying to a sprinter "you should move up in distance" is like saying to a duck, "you should really try bowling."

Runners are the Don Quixotes of the world, forever flailing at windmills, sometimes laughed at, rarely understood.

—Michael Sandrock

Running is such a part of my life. If I were never to run another marathon, I would still do two-hour runs.

—Joan Benoit Samuelson

We're talking about a social movement. It was something that . . . was growing, the idea that you could train at any age, that almost anyone could run a marathon if they ran slow enough, and were patient and drank enough liquid along the way.

—Kenny Moore, on the birth of the running movement in the 1970s

I've always got such high expectations for myself. I'm aware of them, but I can't relax them.

—Mary Decker-Slaney

No other sport is as democratic as running.

—Florence Griffith Joyner and Jon Hanc, *Running for Dummies*

You talk to enough runners, you'll find out how superstitious many of us are.

—Dick Beardsley

Except for .001 percent of the running population, everyone's in the same exact position: There will always be people slower than you, and people faster.

—"Ask Miles," *Runner's World*

That's the thing about running: your greatest runs are rarely measured by racing success. They are moments in time when running allows you to see how wonderful your life is.

—Kara Goucher, elite American long-distance runner who placed third at the 2012 U.S. Olympic marathon trials

Start slowly and taper off.

—Walt Stack, R.I.P.

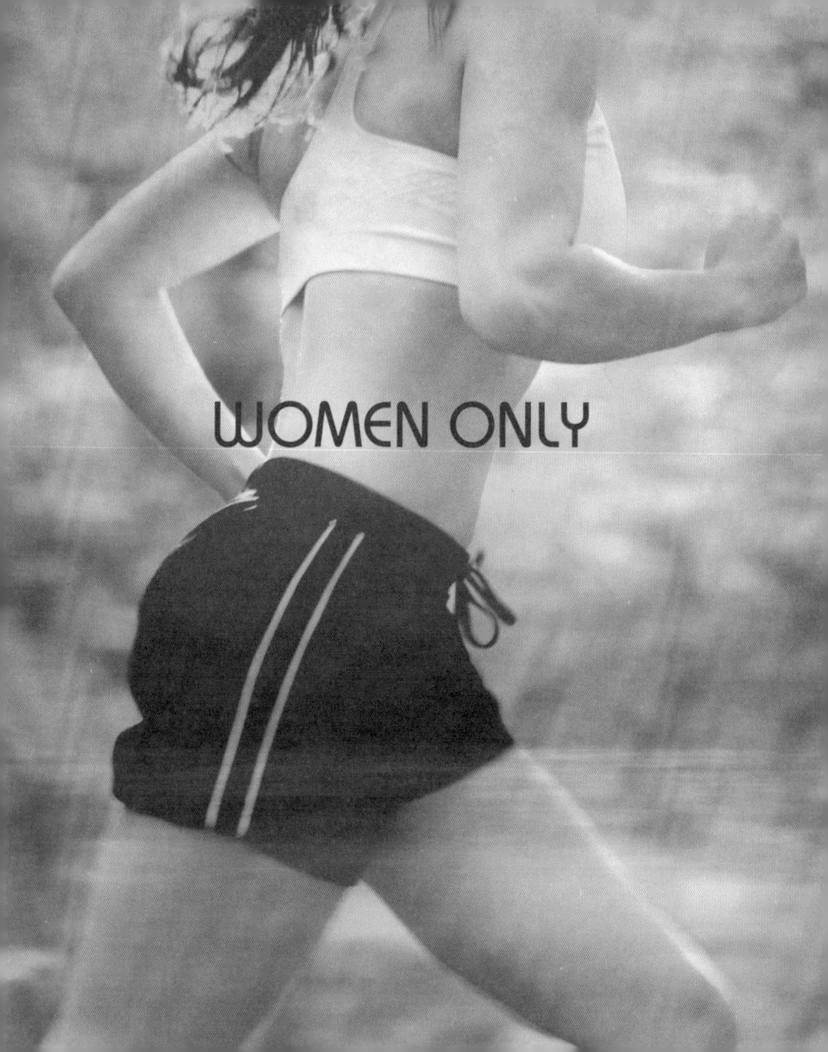
WOMEN ONLY

Several weeks before the start of the 1996 Olympic Games in Atlanta, an essay appeared in the Sunday Magazine of the New York Times *with the headline, "How the Women Won." The piece opened with these two provocative paragraphs:*

> When the modern Olympics began in Athens in 1896, one dismissive tradition carried over from the ancient games. All 245 athletes from 14 nations who competed in Athens were men. Women were expected to lend their applause, not their athletic skills. Olympic historians now believe that two women ran the marathon course near or during the Games. If so, the organizers were unimpressed. Distance running by women was thought to be un-ladylike, a violation of natural law. The common wisdom held that a woman was not physiologically capable of running mile after mile; that she wouldn't be able to bear children; that her uterus would fall out; that she might grow a mustache; that she was a man, or wanted to be one.

When six women collapsed after the 800-meters race at the 1928 Amsterdam Olympics, an alarmist account in The New York Times said that "even this distance makes too great a call on feminine strength." The London Daily Mail carried admonitions from doctors that women who participated in such "feats of endurance" would "become old too soon." The 800-meters race was discontinued. For 32 years, until the 1960 Rome Olympics, women would run no race longer than 200 meters.

That distance restriction eventually changed, but it wasn't easy shaking off tradition's chastity belt. A cabal of old men ran the Olympics. They had even older-fashioned views about women and sports unless it involved "ladylike" activities such as swimming, diving, ice-skating, and gymnastics.

Then along came late-Sixties trailblazers like Kathrine Switzer who ran the Boston Marathon in 1967 when women were officially prohibited. (Women were not allowed to enter the Boston officially until five years later. Switzer competed at Boston six times, finishing second in 1975 in 2:51). Her courageous performance that day opened the door for women distance runners everywhere. The passage of Title IX in 1972 as part of the Education Act—the amendment outlawed gender-based discrimination at colleges that received U.S. Federal funds—kicked that door wide open and led to an explosion of college athletic scholarships for women which, in turn encouraged more girls to play sports in high school.

Women's running benefited. But change didn't happen overnight. It wasn't until 1984 that the women's marathon finally became an officially sanctioned Olympic event. Joan Benoit Samuelson, of Maine, took the gold in that inaugural race in 2:24. In high school, she had who won the 1975 state championship in the mile—the longest distance a high school girl was then allowed to run in a track meet.

Flash forward to the modern running era. At the 2011 Boston Marathon, almost half the field of 24,340 runners was women. Ninety-eight percent of these 10,285 starters completed the 26.2-mile course. At the 2011 Nike Women's Marathon in San Francisco, 4,401 women finished with an average time of 5:09. Women runners now make up 53 percent of all race participants in the U.S. and 41 percent of all marathon finishers.

Back then, women were not supportive of a woman running. Sweating in public was very unfeminine.

—Kathrine Switzer, referring to being a runner in 1967; in 1998 she was one of the five inaugural inductees into the National Distance Running Hall of Fame

Get the hell out of my race and give me that number!

—Boston Marathon race official Jock Semple to Kathrine Switzer, as he tried to yank her off the course before Switzer's boyfriend shoved him aside

I'm not prejudiced against women; they just can't run in my race!

—Jock Semple, on why he tried to prevent Kathrine Switzer from running the Boston Marathon

I started the Boston Marathon as a 20-year-old girl, and came out the other end a grown woman.

—Kathrine Switzer

When I go to the Boston Marathon now, I have wet shoulders—women fall into my arms crying. They're weeping for joy because running has changed their lives. They feel they can do anything.

—Kathrine Switzer

A male runner in distress is a heroic figure; a woman runner in distress is further proof that we are fragile creatures who are physiologically unsuited to marathon running.

—Kathrine Switzer, *Marathon Woman*

Running was in my blood from the beginning. If God has given you a talent, you have to show it. People told me, 'You won't have children if you run long distances.' It was lies. I wanted to be like the men. If no one gives you encouragement, you have to encourage yourself.

—Tegla Loroupe, of Kenya, women's winner of numerous marathons: New York City, London, Boston, Rotterdam, Hong Kong, Berlin and Rome

When it was over, I told [my husband] Scott, "Never again." But then again, I said the same thing after my first marathon.

—Joan Benoit Samuelson, on giving birth to her first child, a daughter

Of all the challenges I have faced, the greatest one has been the quest for combining my family and career.

—Joan Benoit Samuelson

Like so many women, sometimes my needs and interests are congruous, and sometimes they compete with each other for my time, energy, and focus.

—Joan Benoit Samuelson

Leave your watch on the kitchen table and go—freely, like a child.

—Claire Kowalchik, *The Complete Book of Running for Women*

Sex doesn't always determine who will be the fastest. Look at any race and you'll see that the best women beat most of the men.

—Claire Kowalchik

It changed my life enormously. I had my head so firmly planted in the sand. Now I see how flimsy life is.

—Priscilla Welch on her cancer diagnosis

When I was growing up I wasn't inspired to be a marathoner. It wasn't even in a little girl's vocabulary.

—Lorraine Moller

Our headmistress told us not to run cross-country or we'd end up looking like Russian shot putters. I started measuring my legs everyday to see if they were getting too muscular. I decided when they increased above a certain size I'd stop running.

—Lorraine Moller

When I was a little girl, my parents said studying was the most important thing. "You need your job in the future, not sport," they told me. They couldn't believe running would be such a big thing for me.

—Uta Pippig, of Germany, and the first woman to win the Boston Marathon three consecutive times (1994–1996)

I see elegance and beauty in every female athlete. I don't think being an athlete is unfeminine. I think of it as a kind of grace.

—Jackie Joyner-Kersey, winner of three gold Olympic gold medals (heptathlon twice; long jump once)

My parents had a certain idea of what they wanted their little girl to be and it did not include a budding track star.

—Grete Waitz

People used to think I was a freak. Now women of all shapes and sizes run all the time. And they're not just beautiful and slim and wearing pink gossamer tights. They jiggle along at 12-minute miles or spring along at 6:30s. That's what I love.

—Kathrine Switzer

At least in a race you have mile markers and know how long you have to go. Labor is like running as hard as you can without knowing where the finish line is.

—Lorraine Moller on childbirth

I fell in love with the Boston Marathon in 1964. I was running through the woods with the neighborhood dogs when I first saw it. For me, running was a form of communion with nature and a way to rejoin my mind and body. Hardly anyone ran back then. But I just love to run. I didn't know the marathon was closed to women, and I set about training in nurses' shoes with no instructions, no coach and no books. At first, I had no intention of making any kind of statement, I was following my heart for no other reason than I felt moved by some inner force—passion. [In 1966] I wrote for my application to the Boston Athletic Association (BAA). The Boston Marathon was the only marathon I had ever heard of. Will Cloney, the race director, wrote back a letter that said that women were not physiologically capable of running 26 miles and furthermore, under the rules that governed international sports, they were not allowed to run. I was stunned. "All the more reason to run," I thought.

—Roberta Gibb, first woman to "unofficially" run the Boston Marathon

When I am running, I feel everything is in sync. Even my mechanical leg becomes a part of me.

—Sarah Reinersten, raced on the U.S. Disabled Track Team for 10 years, and was first female leg amputee to finish the Hawaii Ironman

So many more girls are involved in sports, it's such a great time for women's sports, we're trying to push it as hard as we can.

—Liz Dolan, Nike's vice president for marketing, told the *New York Times* in 1996

My basic philosophy can be summed up by an expression we use in Norwegian: hurry slowly. Get there, but be patient.

—Grete Waitz

I ran to be free; I ran to avoid pain; I ran to feel pain; I ran out of love and hate and anger and joy.

—Dagny Scott, author of *Runner's World Complete Book of Women's Running*

My first year of running was spent going to road races around the New England area. I was welcomed by my fellow male runners, but often not by race promoters or race officials.

—Charlotte Lettis Richardson, a national caliber runner in the 1970s, she won the L'eggs Mini Marathon in Central Park in New York City

In 1970 when I started running there were very few opportunities for women runners to compete at longer distances. We could run the 880 and the mile, but not much further.

—Charlotte Lettis Richardson

Years ago, women sat in kitchens drinking coffee and discussing life. Today, they cover the same topics while they run.

—Joan Benoit Samuelson

Gazelles run when they're pregnant. Why should it be any different for women?

—Joan Ullyot, M.D.

When I started running after the birth of my daughter, I had over 50 pounds to lose. What helped me greatly was constant positive reinforcement. I didn't think of myself as a fat runner because I knew that such negative thinking wasn't going to help me to lose the weight.

—Florence Griffith Joyner

The history of women's competitive racing can be traced back to ancient Greece, when every five years a short footrace was held at a women's festival to honor the Greek goddess Hera.

—Shanti Sosienski, *Women Who Run*

Running is my meditation, mind flush, cosmic telephone, mood elevator, and spiritual communion.

—Lorraine Moller

Do the work. Do the analysis. But feel your run. Feel your race. Feel the joy that is running.

—Kara Goucher

As I approach my non-racing future, I realize that running is its own reward. It's not the calories burned, or the awards received, or the free shoes from New Balance, or the money, or the records, or the magazine interviews, or even the lifelong friendships—though all of those are wonderful—but running itself that gets me out of the door day in and day out. I can honestly say I couldn't live without running. I could exist, yes, but not live.

—Joan Nesbit Mabe, in a *Running Times* interview in 2002

There are two rules: You have to be a mom (people ask if adopting a baby counts, and I say, "yes, of course"); and you have to be able to run three miles without stopping.

—Joan Nesbit Mabe, on being a coach for See Jane Run, a mothers' running group

I always loved running... it was something you could do by yourself, and under your own power. You could go in any direction, fast or slow as you wanted, fighting the wind if you felt like it, seeking out new sights just on the strength of your feet and the courage of your lungs.

—Paula Radcliffe

[W]omen like Olympian Paula Radcliffe have world record marathon times that are sub-2:20—that's more than two hours faster than the first woman known to run a marathon in 1896.

—Shanti Sosienski, author of *Women Who Run*

When you have the enthusiasm and the passion, you end up figuring how to excel.

—Deena Kastor, selected as the top women's marathoner in the world in 2006 by *Track and Field News* magazine

We make choices. I hate to say 'sacrifices.' When I speak to younger groups, to colleges and other younger athletes, I say 'we don't make sacrifices. If we truly love this sport and we have these goals and dreams in the sport, the classroom, or in life, they're not sacrifices. They're choices that we make to fulfill these goals and dreams.' Sacrifices makes it sound like "Oh, poor me, I have to do this in order to get to this," and I don't really like that word. It was just really the choice to take care of myself and live a proper lifestyle.

—Deena Kastor

You know, I'm no women's libber, but the media can really irritate me. I sure get tired of being "pert" Francie Larrieu. That kind of stuff has to stop. All those ridiculous adjectives they use with women.

—Francie Larrieu, a five-time Olympian, started running at age 13 and ran for the San Jose Cindergals, one of the first youth track clubs for women

The Zulu warrior women could run fifty miles a day and fight at the end of it. Fifty miles together, perfectly in step, so the veldt drummed with it. Did their hearts beat as one? My heart can beat with theirs, slow and strong and efficient—pumping energy.

—Sara Maitland, author of "The Loveliness of the Long-Distance Runner"

If this race is for "men only," why doesn't it say "men only" on the entry blank?

—Nina Kuscsik in 1969; she won both the Boston and New York City Marathons in 1972

Once I was out for a twenty-miler on the grass along the Parkway, but I was picked up by the police after three miles. It was raining and someone called and told them 'There's a crazy woman running . . ..' They took me and left me off at the next exit.

—Nina Kuscsik, on running in the 1960s

Running is the space in my day when I feel the most beautiful—when I don't feel judged by others. And that's what I want for all little girls.

—Molly Barker, founder of Girls on the Run International

When the desire strikes, simply put on a pair of shorts and a T-shirt, lace up your running shoes, and head down the road, up a trail, or through an open field.

—Claire Kowalchik

Just like I hope to be a mother the rest of my life, I hope to be a runner the rest of my life.

—Joan Benoit Samuelson

We've suffered the pain, felt the glory, and, when all the sweat is spent, we have the faith to reach deep inside to find that ounce of energy left in our heels, our heart, our soul, to carry us across the finish line stiff-legged and fatigue-racked, but with a smile of victory.

—Gail W. Kislevitz

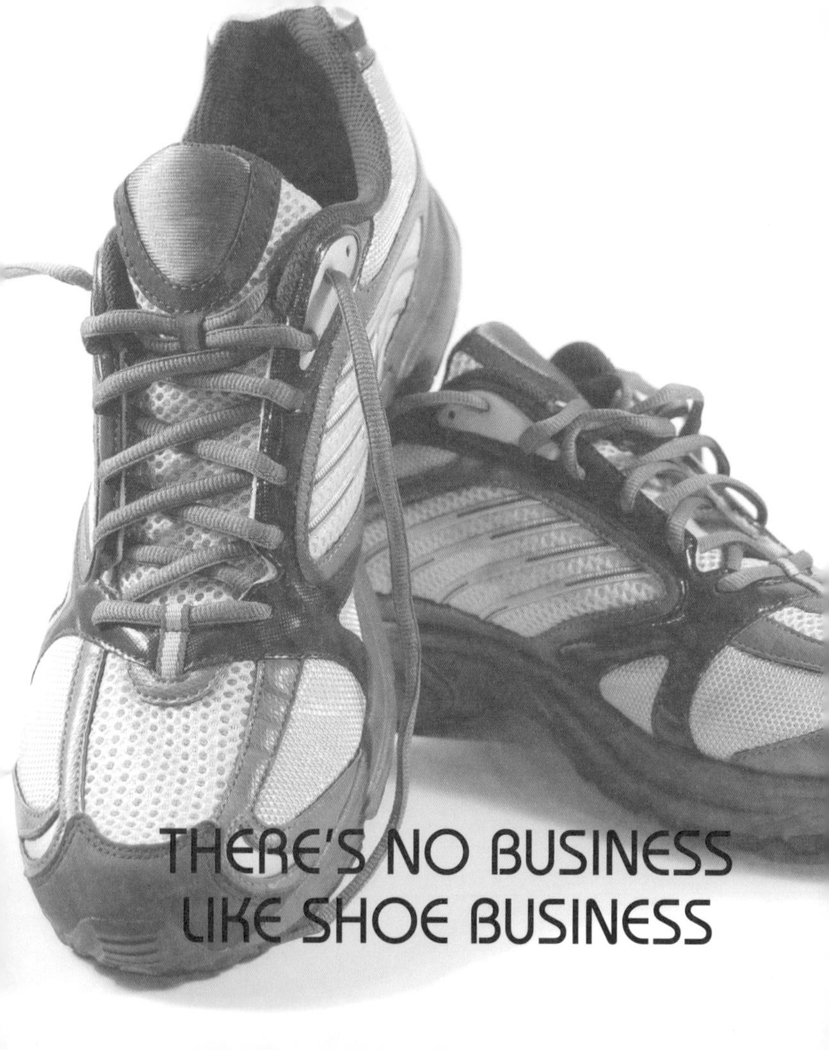
THERE'S NO BUSINESS
LIKE SHOE BUSINESS

Compared to other sports, running can be done on the cheap, which is an appealing quality in difficult economic times. A pair of shoes is the only significant investment required, unless you prefer barefoot running — which is preferred by fewer than 1% of all runners in the United States.

Because most runners tend to be obsessive about what they put on their feet, they are highly opinionated when it comes to footwear. The average runner purchases three pairs of running shoes each year. A runner's closet is often overflowing with old and new shoes, reminding him or her of all the mileage spent in them.

The multi-billion dollar athletic footwear industry constantly stokes our hunger for new shoe models and brands. No one is spared this commercial onslaught. Whether you're a veteran marathoner or 5K first-timer, you're often at the mercy of the great footwear powers who might inexplicably discontinue a favorite model.

These days, buying a new pair of running shoes seems to require advanced degrees in podiatry, biomechanics and material sciences. Of course, if the shoe fits . . .

The hottest new footwear trend is minimalism that

echoes running shoes from the late 1960s and early 70s — lightweight, flat soles, thin tread, little cushioning or arch support, and no built-up heel. When the running boom swelled the ranks of joggers and recreational runners into the millions, athletic footwear companies like Nike, Asics, New Balance, and Adidas answered their needs with built-up shoes offering the latest in comfort, cushioning, and support. It turned into an R&D arms race for feet. But here comes the shocker: injury rates have remained virtually the same for runners over the past 40 years.

So have we then come full-circle with minimalist running shoes? That less *shoe is better than more shoe? The jury is still out whether minimalism is here to stay, or is even and safe and appropriate for certain kinds of injury-prone runners. Bottom line: who knows what running shoes will look like three or five years from now?*

A runner's two greatest loyalties are not to any shoe company or model, but to the left foot and the right.

—Joe Henderson

I believe in gradual experimentation with running shoes.

—Bill Rodgers

I believe in keeping running simple and, in regard to shoes, that would mean no gimmicks, unnecessary cushioning, etc.

—Bill Rodgers

Sometimes . . . an injury may be due to increased running, fatigue, sickness, etc. and have nothing at all to do with your shoe.

—Bill Rodgers

No doubt a brain and some shoes are essential for marathon success, although if it comes down to a choice, pick the shoes. More people finish marathons with no brains than with no shoes.

—Don Kardong, author, journalist, coach, fourth-place finisher at the Montreal Olympic marathon

When I was about 14 or 15, and running in a pretty muddy cross country race, one of my shoes stuck in the mud and came off. Boy, was I wild. To think that I had trained hard for this race and didn't do up my shoelace tightly enough! I really got aggressive with myself, and I found myself starting to pass a lot of runners. As it turned out, I improved something like twenty places in that one race. But I never did get my shoe back.

—Rob de Castella, won the 1981 Fukuoka Marathon in a world-record time of 2:08:18

Running shoes may be the most destructive force to ever hit the human foot.

—Christopher McDougall

One surprising advantage the Tarahumara seem to have over the rest of the world is their lack of technology. They essentially run barefoot or in sandals and experience very little in the way of injury. Over the years, running shoes have become more and more cushioned with more and more high-tech gadgetry attached. Rather than improving our runs, these developments seem to have worsened them. The latest gotta-have running shoe in the stores is causing the average runner to land in a continuous unnatural position, causing more harm over the long haul than good. I can say, as someone who's run many a marathon in little more than canvas and rubber, that there is some truth to this. Like the rest of our bodies, the foot is designed to run. Simplicity is key. A shoe shouldn't be a La-Z-Boy recliner.

—Bill Rodgers, reviewing *Born to Run* for the *San Francisco Chronicle*

Shoes do no more for the foot than a hat does for the brain.

—Dr. Mercer Rang, orthopedic surgeon and researcher in pediatric development

The ideal shoe would provide enough support for a runner during a race, but would fall apart once that runner crossed the finish line.

—Bill Bowerman

The ordinary track shoe is covered with junk. Leather trim, tongue, laces. All unnecessary.

—Bill Bowerman, from *Sports Illustrated* profile in 1960

These Cortez Shoes know all the hard times that we had been through
All the craziest things we used to do just to get by walk in my shoes and you
Will see why these Cortez shoes try n walk in these Cortez shoes betcha couldn't
Walk in a mile in these shoes but we get by and we got to keep on walkin."

—chorus part from "Cortez Shoes," by Lil Rob, a Mexican-American music producer and rapper, in 2008

Sellers of running shoes love us runners. We're quick to buy a shoe in the belief that it can make us healthier.

—Joe Henderson, writer, coach, and prolific author of running books

The longer we run in a certain shoe, the stronger the attachment to it and the greater the sense of loss when this pair wears out and can't be replaced. At rare times when they do, this model often has changed or disappeared before we can replace the original.

—Joe Henderson

Your spikes, which were really quite long then, would catch the material of the track and your shoe would get heavier. I was simply filing them down and rubbing some graphite on the spikes. I thought I would run more effectively.

—Roger Bannister

Maybe wearing heavy boots in training and light shoes in competition was good; when you change, whoosh. It was very practical.

—Emil Zatopek on wearing Czech army-issue military boots in training

I run and run, soft and squishy, easy rhythm, thinking of other things, and [my wife] Dana comes home and there is yelling. Soapsuds down the hall! Soapsuds in my kitchen! But even she admit no one ever got shirts so white!

—Emil Zatopek, on doing laundry by putting it in the bathtub with soap and water, putting on combat boots, and running in place on the clothes

If you want shoes with lots of pep, get Keds. For bounce and zoom in every step, get Keds.

—Kedso the Clown, from 1963 Keds television commercial

I would advise that each runner leave shoes and stockings at home, but of course this should be optional with the individual; next to bare feet are sandals, next to sandals moccasins, next to moccasins, soft, low shoes.

—J. William Lloyd, who in 1890 wrote the first treatise on running

Blaming the running injury epidemic on big, bad Nike seems too easy—but that's okay, because it's largely their fault.

—Christopher McDougall

Our search for elusive, and probably unattainable, perfection resumes. You know you're a real runner when you have stocked a closet with failed shoes, with hundreds of unrun miles still in them.

—Joe Henderson

Motion-controlled shoes and orthotics are like putting a cast on a broken limb. The pain may stop, but the longer you use it, the weaker you get.

—Steve Sashen

Shoe monogamy is vastly overrated. The first time is always the best with your new pair of running shoes.

—Bill Katovsky

Even if shoes could be perfect, we can't. Our biomechanical oddities and running excesses cause most of our troubles. Even the best shoes can't overcome these imperfections and indiscretions.

—Joe Henderson

Each time you try on a pair of shoes, find a hard surface to walk on rather than the thick soft carpet in shoe stores, where almost any shoe will feel good. If there's no sturdy floor to walk on, ask if you can walk outside (if you're not allowed, shop elsewhere).

—Dr. Phil Maffetone, *The Big Book of Endurance Training and Racing*

Abandon the notion that you have a *shoe size*. Instead you have a *foot size*. Shoes are made all over the world and apply different shapes and standards.

—Dr. Mark Cucuzzella, owner of Two Rivers Treads, the nation's first minimalist shoe store

I see shoes as tools.

—Angie Hotz, aka "Barefoot Angie Bee" and run coach

There's never quite the perfect shoe. It's a quest. In 1976 I did have a pair of running shoes from Asics, I wish they still made them, the Asics Montreal. They were phenomenal shoes. They were light, they didn't wear down fast, great shoe, fit perfect. They were the best shoes I ever wore.

—Bill Rodgers, in 2009 *New York Times* interview

Nike actually got it right with its first few generations of shoes. They were thin and light, offering just what runners needed and no more: a little protection from rough ground and cold weather. But problems arise when protection turns into correction, and marketing takes over for education. Once gimmicks take over and technique is scuttled, you can expect up to 90 percent of all marathon runners to become injured.

—Christopher McDougall

There is an expression among even the most advanced runners that getting your shoes on is the hardest part of any workout.

—Kathrine Switzer

My first running shoes from 1970 were leather moccasins I purchased on a Native American reservation. Best shoes I ever owned.

—Scott Tinley, two-time winner of Hawaii Ironman Triathlon

I know guys who can run marathons but can't sprint to anyone's rescue unless they put their shoes on first.

—Erwan Le Corre

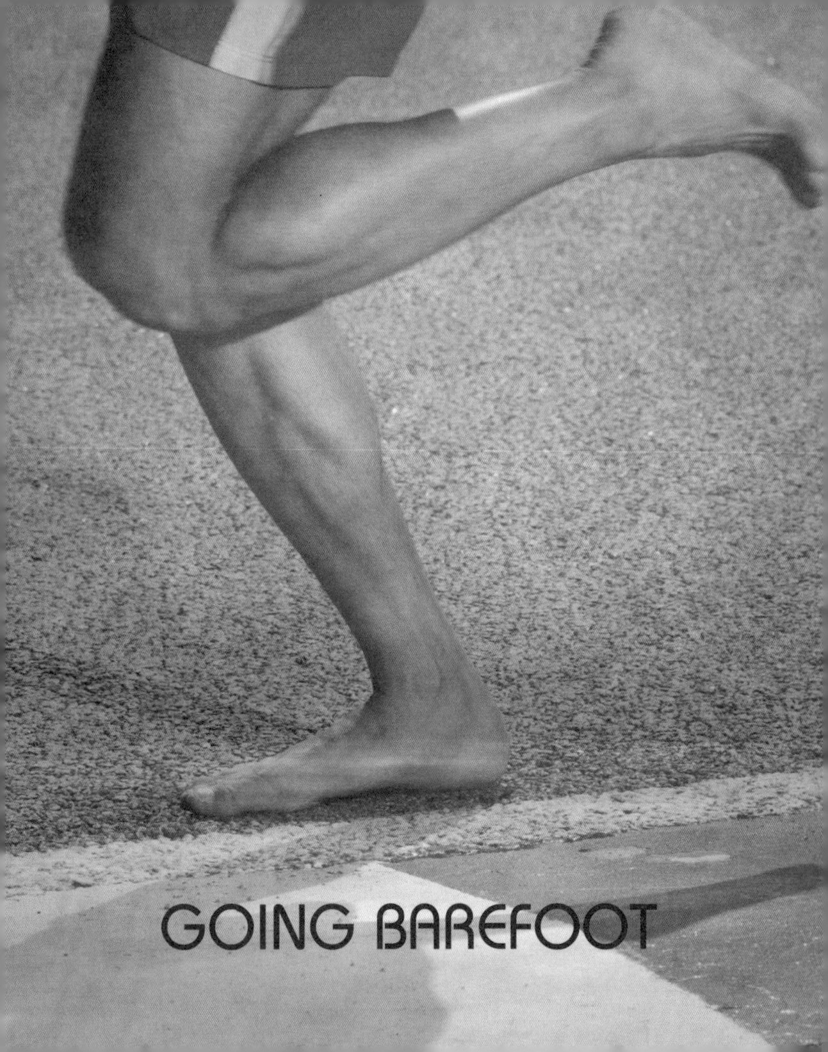
GOING BAREFOOT

Barefoot running gets plenty of media attention these days; so, one should expect to see a lot more unshod half-marathoners and marathoners. Yet, in big-city races, just a handful of barefoot runners will brave 26.2 miles of asphalt in Boston, New York City or Chicago. The reason why? Old habits die slowly. Millions of runners' feet have been spoiled, pampered, and coddled in over-supported shoes ever since the running revolution first took flight during the late Sixties.

That decade began, curiously enough, with a barefoot bias among a distinguished roster of champion runners. We all know about Abebe Bikila whose bare feet flew over the cobblestones en route to winning the marathon at the 1960 Rome Olympics. (The Ethiopian runner wasn't the first marathoner to go barefoot in the Olympics—that honor belongs to a tribesman from South Africa named Len Tau who finished ninth at the St. Louis Games in 1904.) Fewer of us are probably familiar with the serial accomplishments of Herb Elliott, a talented, Australian middle-distance runner who appeared twice on the cover of Sports Illustrated, *in 1958 and 1960, both times running barefoot!*

Elliott trained barefoot with runs along the beach and sandy dunes. He also held the world record in the mile

(3:54), and at the Rome Games, he won the gold medal in the 1,500 meters and bettered his own world record with a time of 3:35.6.

Known as "Europe's Barefoot Champion," England's Bruce Tulloh won the European 5,000 meters championship in 1962 by racing unshod on the cinder track. Tulloh had started running barefoot three years earlier because he was convinced that shoes were slowing him down. In short order and without shoes cramping his style, Tulloh won his first British amateur title barefoot and continued racing and setting U.K. records, including the two miles in 8:34, until he retired from competition in 1967. (Two years later, he ran across the U.S. in 64 days, but with shoes, due to his uncertainty about road conditions.)

Going barefoot was also popular among other elite British runners, such as Ron Hill, who ran unshod when he took second in the International Cross-Country Championship in 1964. At the Mexico Olympics, he placed seventh in the 10,000 meters, again without shoes. Hill recently told Running Times, *"I was going to run the marathon at the 1972 Munich Olympics barefoot, but the Germans laid new stone chippings on parts of the course."*

Yet when we think of contemporary barefoot runners, one of the first who comes to mind is Zola Budd, who inadvertently played a game of Twister with Mary Decker in the 3,000-meters finals at the 1984 Los Angeles Olympics. That track incident severely dampened the public's enthusiasm for barefoot running. So it went into deep hibernation, only to energetically emerge from its shoeless slumber nearly 25 years later with the runaway success of the national bestseller Born to Run. *But author Christopher McDougall remains a modest fellow who deliberately avoids taking much of the credit for unleashing the barefoot dogs of footwear. In a 2010 interview for Zero-Drop.com, he said, "I'm the showboat son who arrives late to the party and pretends he threw it."*

Then let's hear from some of the other Sole Train party guests.

Shoes have technology to cushion you and absorb force, but when you run barefoot, you have to run gently and lightly. It's farcical to believe that barefoot running's a fad, because we've been running for millions of years and didn't need shoes and Gatorade when we started. I'm not sure it's doing us that much good.

—Daniel Lieberman

Coming from a farming background, I saw nothing out of the ordinary in running barefoot, although it seemed to startle the rest of the athletics world. I have always enjoyed going barefoot and when I was growing up I seldom wore shoes, even when I went into town.

—Zola Budd, twice broke the world record in the women's 5,000 meters

I found [shoes] uncomfortable and after that I decided to continue running barefoot because I found it more comfortable. I felt more in touch with what was happening. I could actually feel the track.

—Zola Budd

They were the lightest shoes I could find.

—Ron Hill, elite British long-distance runner, on why he ran barefoot

There are many ways to run other than barefoot. For example, without shoes, shoeless, unshod, or devoid of footwear.

—Steven Sashen

People [say to] me after a race, "I get so many blisters from shoes, if I run barefoot, it's going to be worse." And I say, "Well that's why I stopped wearing shoes because I got tired of getting blisters."

—Ken Bob Saxton, aka "Barefoot Ken Bob," has run 76 marathons, 75 of them shoeless, since 1997

Personally, I found it strange that so many people have never tried running barefoot, and some even act as if running barefoot were the most unnatural thing in the universe!

—Barefoot Ken Bob

My journey of discovery began afar: while watching Kenyan runners go barefoot. I applied this natural way of running to my own jogging. I learned how to run softly.

—Mark Cucuzzella, M.D.

I now do almost all my running barefoot on pavement and grass surfaces. I use shoes for races and longer and quicker road work. It is almost impossible to hurt yourself running barefoot on hard surface if you use your brain. You self-regulate in a way you cannot when in shoes. You land soft and if something shows even the slightest discomfort you stop.

—Mark Cucuzzella, M.D.

I've never seen a barefoot kid running around and playing voluntarily in summer and have an overuse injury.

—Mark Cucuzzella, M.D.

The foot can return 70 percent of its energy. I'm waiting for the perfect shoe that can do better.

—Mark Cucuzzella, M.D.

The shoemaker's children go barefoot.

—Danish proverb

No elite runner today would compete barefoot, and I don't blame them. If my entire livelihood were hanging in the balance, I wouldn't risk stepping on a bottle cap 50 yards from the finish line. But let's keep in mind that pro runners are wearing only the thinnest, lightest shoes available. They would never wear the kind of motion-controlling, super-cushioned foamboats that *Runner's World* is constantly pimping in their shoe review issues. They already know how to run barefoot-style, so all they want is some protection for their soles, just like the Tarahumara with their huaraches and Apaches with their moccasins. The goal isn't to run barefoot—the goal is to learn to run properly, and bare feet are the most effective and trustworthy method.

—Christopher McDougall

Going Barefoot

People laughed at me. There were acorns on the course. Those guys thought I was absolutely crazy. They said, 'Man, you're going to hurt your feet." Didn't bother me at all.

—Dale Story, a junior at Oregon State won the 1961 NCAA cross-country championship by running barefoot

In essence, the human foot behaves like a spring, capable of storing and returning up to 70 percent of the energy that goes into it. Running shoes do not even come close to this figure.

—Dr. Michael Yessis, author of *Explosive Running*

I can't prove this, but I believe when my runners train barefoot, they run faster and suffer fewer injuries.

—Vin Lananna, Director of Track and Field for the University of Oregon and seven-time NCAA Coach of the Year, from www.chrismcdougall.com/blog

All the [Kenyan] children are running barefoot. It's interesting to note that here the only children wearing running shoes are at the very back of the field. In one race, the further back in the field the girls finish, the better their shoes, to the absurd extent that the girl with the newest, sleekest running shoes of all comes in last, while the girl whose shoes are only slightly worse finishes second to last. Ironically, the prize for the winner in each race is a pair of Nike running trainers.

—Adharanand Finn, from his book *Running with the Kenyans*, describing a local inter-schools cross-country race

As a kid who couldn't yet find good shoes, I ran barefoot whenever the weather and surface allowed — and was never healthier. Next I ran mainly in flimsy racing shoes, and finally in bulkier models. The trend toward more and more of a shoe parallels my trend toward more and more injuries.

—Joe Henderson

There are evolutionary biologists who make a strong argument that we evolved to run, thus it may be the most natural way to exercise. However, along with me, up to 50 to 75 percent of runners sustain some type of injury in a given year. That seems unnatural if we truly evolved to run. I am now running barefoot 20 miles per week without any hip or other problems, despite being 30 years older.

—Dr. Irene Davis, director of the Spaulding National Running Center at Harvard Medical School

We found pockets of people all over the globe who are still running barefoot, and what you find is that during propulsion and landing, they have far more range of motion in the foot and engage more of the toe. Their feet flex, spread, splay and grip the surface, meaning you have less pronation and more distribution of pressure.

—Jeff Pisciotta, Senior Researcher, Nike's Sports Research Lab, from www.chrismcdougall.com/blog

Barefoot Shoes: the running world's homage to Orwell.

—Josh Sutcliffe, aka "Barefoot Josh"

Barefoot running is not simply running, except without the shoes. Do not try to learn barefoot running in minimalist footwear. Do not confuse barefoot running with running in "barefoot" shoes —they are as different as night and day, blindfolded and clear-sighted, senseless and sensible. We were blessed with sensitive soles for the same reason we don't like to hold our hand in the fire for long. It hurts to do stupid things.

—Barefoot Ken Bob

Running barefoot on gravel trails was my graduate school.

—Barefoot Ken Bob

Education: what I call "stepping on a rock."

—Barefoot Josh

I encourage people to become more like children. Do not commit yourself to X number of miles, or X number of minutes [of barefoot running]. Instead, try having fun, playing, experimenting, and listening to your bare soles. Children take a few steps, and fall down, and are excited that they took a few steps. Children aren't wondering when they'll be able to run their next marathon!

—Barefoot Ken Bob

One cannot abruptly make the change to being barefoot after years of wearing dangerous footwear: those thick, over-supported shoes that ruin your feet have also weakened your foot muscles.

—Dr. Phil Maffetone

Our feet must last a lifetime. They're subjected to more wear and tear than any other body part. Just walking a mile, you generate more than sixty tons—that's over 120,000 pounds—of stress on each foot! Fortunately, our feet are actually made to handle such natural stress. It's only when we interfere with nature that problems arise. Almost all foot problems can be prevented, and those that do arise can most often be treated conservatively through self-care by being barefoot.

—Dr. Phil Maffetone

Dirty feet: a fact of life, treated with intense uranium-based anti-fungal creams, radiation, and sandblasting for shoe wearers. Barefooters only need a bar of soap.

— Barefoot Josh

There is nothing that "prepares" you for being barefoot. Nothing. Anything that you put on your feet will change either your stride and biomechanics or the amount of sensation you're feeling in your feet (or both) compared to being barefoot. Take off your shoes, and find the hardest and smoothest surface you can find (like a bike path or street) and run. But only do it for about 200 yards. Then see how you feel the next day.

—Steven Sashen

I got [knee and leg] injuries in college from overtraining. I found it harder and harder to run. I have always loved to run. It got to a point where I couldn't even run one mile without pain. My current running shoes needed to be replaced, but I just didn't want to buy another pair of running shoes. That did not seem to be the answer. I did a lot of research on the Internet about barefoot running. One day, I said to my husband, "What would you think if I ran barefoot?" He said, "Go for it! Give it a try." I did. It worked. I started a little at a time every other day. Slowly built up my mileage. That was three years ago.

—Theresa Withee, aka "Barefoot Mama," 44, mother of three, went 4:01 in the 2011 Boston Marathon

Want to watch a real barefoot runner get a wistful look in his eye? Mention a freshly painted white line on the side of the road. Running on those is just dreamy.

—Steven Sashen

I read everything I could find on the topic. After walking barefoot around the house and around the block for a few days, I went on my first barefoot hike and run. It was a joyous and liberating experience. No braces. No shoes. Just my bare feet against the earth. My hiking and running speed in the beginning was slow and the distances were short as my body slowly rebuilt and learned how to run and walk the way our ancestors have for millions of years. I experienced typical lower calf pain and some blisters the first few weeks, but these disappeared as the feet and legs grew stronger. The stride was shorter and quicker. The feet landed gently and fully on the ground with the balls landing first and with no push-off. The constant lift, bent knees, and the fluid, gentle, no-impact motion of the barefoot landing with the arches and calves acting as natural shock absorbers, lent itself to no joint pain, no ankles sprains, no knee pain, no plantar fasciitis, reduced back pain, and no shoulder pain. The beauty of barefoot running and hiking was that it enforced perfect form. If you were doing it wrong, your body would tell you.

—Glen Raines, aka "Barefoot Caveman", went 3.39 in the 2011 Boston Marathon, from Barefoot Running Society's website

Some doctors like to joke, "Keep up this barefoot running thing... it's putting my kids through college!" They forget that, 40 years ago, doctors made the same joke about running shoes.

—Steven Sashen

When I was 14 or 15, my brother tried to encourage me by giving me a pair of running shoes. But I threw them away because I was so used to running with bare feet and they were too heavy.

—Haile Gebrselassie, Ethiopian running great and former world record holder in the marathon

Going Barefoot

I prefer running without shoes. My toes didn't get cold. Besides, if I'm in front from the start, no one can step on them.

—Michelle Dekkers, the barefoot South African runner who won the 1989 NCAA cross-country title for Indiana University

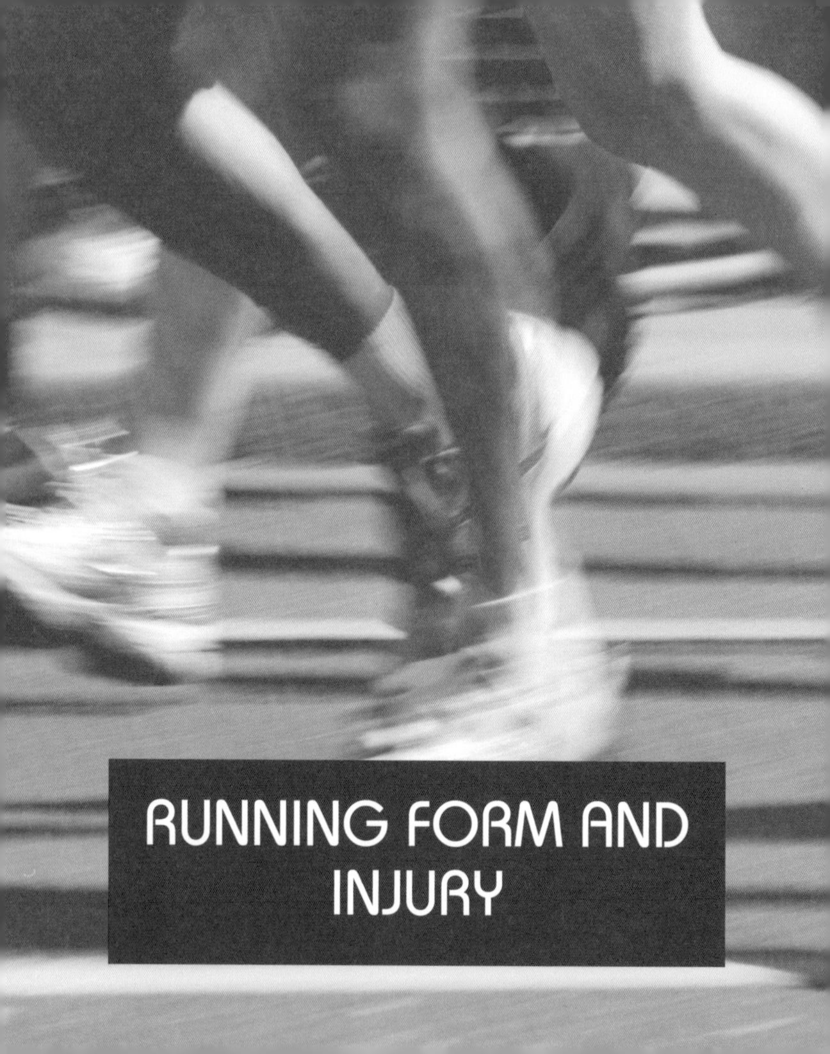

RUNNING FORM AND INJURY

Running Form and Injury

Every runner wants to look and feel good running. The elite distance runners from East Africa make the act of rapidly putting one foot in front of the other seem so maddeningly simple and effortless. Watching these runners get through a full marathon at a sub-five-minutes-per-mile pace is truly awe-inspiring. Their limbs are propelled forward with pure natural ease and balletic grace. They are Nureyevs in Nikes, Baryshnikovs in Brooks. They are born and bred to run.

Aesthetics aside, ideal running form is a result of good biomechanics—of getting the most efficiency out of your body. Poor biomechanics, on the other hand, can lead to reduced power, declining performance, and chronic injury. A faulty gait can also be symptomatic of hidden physical causes with the body trying to overcompensate for a particular dysfunction. For example, a tight left hamstring might be the result of an imbalance in the right foot due to the running shoe not fitting properly.

"An injury is, with some exceptions, simply an end result of a series of dominoes falling over," says Dr. Phil Maffetone, author of The Big Book of Health and Fitness. *"One little, innocuous problem affects something else, and the dominoes start to fall. The end result is, sometimes after*

a half-dozen or so dominoes have fallen, a symptom—pain, dysfunction, loss of power—all depending on how the body adapts and compensates to the falling dominoes."

Proper running form is like learning any athletic skill. It needs to develop over time, but you can expect injury-free, positive results if your body is not pre-occupied with fighting against itself. Of course, there are the rare exceptions like legendary long-distance runner Emil Zatopek who was known as the "Czech Express." The humble, stoop-shouldered, perpetual running machine often trained in heavy combat boots. One hundred-mile training weeks were the norm. Zatopek set 18 world records and is best known for his gold-medal "hat trick" (5,000 meters, 10,000 meters and marathon) at the 1952 Helsinki Olympic Games—a feat never matched.

[Emil Zatopek] ran like a man with a noose around his neck... the most frightful horror spectacle since Frankenstein...on the verge of strangulation; his hatchet face was crimson; his tongue lolled out.

—*New York Herald Tribune* sports columnist Red Smith

[Zatopek] runs like a man who has just been stabbed in the heart.

—European coach

He ran as if his next step would be his last.

—Newspaper account of Emil Zatopek

I shall learn to have a better style once they start judging races according to their beauty. So long as it's a question of speed then my attention will be directed to seeing how fast I can cover the ground.

—Emil Zatopek on his running style

I'm not talented enough to run and smile at the same time.

—Emil Zatopek

We have a magnificent motor at our disposal, but we no longer know how to use it.

—Emil Zatopek

Most runners want to run either longer or faster at some point in their running career, but without good running form, added distance will only lengthen the time you are running improperly and increase your odds of getting hurt.

—George Xu , T'ai Chi Master

It is better, I think, to begin easily and get your running to be smooth and relaxed and then to go faster and faster.

—Henry Rono, three-time NCAA cross-country champion

Run softly by imagining a helium balloon attached to your head.

—Lieutenant Colonel (Dr.) Dan Kuland, U.S. Air Force Chief of Health Promotion

Imagine running on hot coals with a quick cadence.

—Lieutenant Colonel (Dr.) Dan Kuland,

Imagine being reeled in on a big fishing line attached at your belly button.

—Lieutenant Colonel (Dr.) Dan Kuland

If you stand broken, you run broken. Fix your posture, fix your muscles, and fix your running.

—Jay Dicharry, Director of the SPEED Performance Clinic and the Motion Analysis Lab Coordinator at the University of Virginia

Keep those hip flexors supple! You run by storing elastic energy during the loading phase, and then releasing is during propulsion.

—Jay Dicharry

Better skills = better performance. Athletes move dynamically. Runners move repetitively. If you do the same thing over and over again, you get bad at doing everything else. One day a week, do something to work on other aspects of athletic skill that you don't get running. Hop on a rocker board or Swiss ball, or better yet, go skateboard, surf, or ski. Get out of your comfort zone!

—Jay Dicharry

I'm more interested in the future of running form. I couldn't care less what people wear [on their feet]; I'm more concerned about what they do. For too long, all we've heard about is what to buy. What's been missing from the conversation has been how to run properly. I'm convinced that the next big wave in running won't be footwear, but a surge in running coaches who teach proper, gentle, barefoot-style form.

—Christopher McDougall

Our brains have an amazing ability to create a 'cognitive map' of our surroundings. When running, we're able to map out the nuances of the terrain anywhere from several feet to a hundred yards in front of us. With practice, you will begin to develop 'eye-foot' coordination that allows you to instantly find the best spot to place each step. Since I began barefoot and minimalist-shoe running, I have not experienced the bane of trail runners: twisted ankles.

—Jason Robillard, author of *The Barefoot Running Book,* and editor and founder of The Barefoot Running University website

You're only a hamstring injury away from oblivion.

—Steve Jones, just after setting the world record in the marathon

I'm just lucky in terms of the biomechanics.

—Bill Rodgers

The day I see my dog holding a stretch is the day I'll start stretching too.

—Dr. Steve Gangemi, aka "Sock Doc"

Flexibility is a reflection of overall health and fitness. Stretching does absolutely nothing for health or fitness. It's not exercise. It's not a warm-up or a cool-down. And it definitely doesn't substitute for restful sleep or a wholesome diet.

—Dr. Steve Gangemi

I realized he had talent. We'd go out on runs, and I had to work hard, concentrate on every stride. Bill would float along, with that vacant look in his eyes.

—Amby Burfoot, on his Wesleyan College roommate Bill Rodgers

It was his relaxation that most amazed me. He seemed to be able to run with almost complete detachment from the mental and physical effort involved.

—Amby Burfoot, on Bill Rodgers

He runs with the grace of a bag thrown off the back of a mail truck. Somehow he finds the will to win.

—Hal Higdon, on Alberto Salazar

The fact is, shoes are only a small part of the story of injury-prevention. What is most important is your technique. That has to be learned and practiced. This is really the best insurance against any running injuries in your future.

—Danny Dreyer, author and co-founder of ChiRunning

When I returned to running over 14 years ago, I ran in traditional bulky heeled shoes just like most people. Luckily, I never had a serious injury but I had mediocre finishing times and long recoveries. Despite my high level of training and poor times, I began to research the differences in the elite runners and myself. I found that most of the elite guys were running in less heel lift shoes therefore making them land with a mid-foot strike. I adopted a natural running gait that took me off of my heels, therefore, bettering my race times from the marathon to 24-hour distances. My recovery time also improved to nearly a quarter of the time it had when I was in traditional shoes.

—Rick Meyers, an ultra-runner and owner of The Runner's Sole, a running specialty store in Chambersburg, Pennsylvania

The laws of gravity seemingly don't apply to top runners. These athletically gifted sprites must have secret jet packs.

—Bill Katovsky

Proprioception is the body's awareness of its own motion and position. It's essential to enjoyable and injury-free running and is the secret to optimum performance. Understanding and developing your proprioceptive sense is the first step on the journey towards awakening the skill of natural movement.

—Lee Saxby, British running coach

Running should be tap, tap, tap....not thud, thud, thud.

—Mark Cucuzzella, M.D.

The Tarahumara Indians run in a style reflective of how we all ran as children; they land lightly on their mid-foot (not the heel), have a slight forward lean, and are completely relaxed and happy.

—Mark Cucuzzella, M.D.

A runner will typically average 1,200 steps a mile on one foot. And the gravity force on the body structure is 2.5 times the body weight with each step in the mid-stance phase of gait, no matter if you are running in perfect Kenyan style or in the heel-strike "jogging" pattern.

—Mark Cucuzzella, M.D.

Sometimes the difference between a good and a great runner is only an inch, as measured by exercise scientists. A good runner lifts two inches off the ground with each stride. A great runner rises only one inch, thus conserves energy.

—Hal Higdon

[Roger] Bannister had terrific grace, a terrific long stride, he seemed to ooze power. It was as if the Greeks had come back and brought him to show you what the true Olympic runner was like.

—*Daily Mail* journalist Terry O'Connor

Stop bouncing, and you'll knock twenty seconds off.

—Secretary of the British Olympic Association's advice to Bannister when he ran a mile in 4:52 in his freshman year at Oxford

I knew I had it in me but I had to prove it to myself. Now I'm ready to run with anybody cause I know what I can take I'll just have to polish up on my form which was not the best but not bad either.

—Steve Prefontaine in a 1969 letter

His talent was not that he had great style. He didn't. It got better, I think. We worked probably harder on that than we did on anything.

—Walt McClure, who was Steve Prefontaine's high school coach

Ten Easy-to-Remember "Pearls" for Good Running Form

1. Use quick cadence or leg turnover, but do not shorten your stride. With proper hip extension the stride is actually longer by forward spring.

2. Land lightly on the middle portion of your foot—not the heels, or toes like a sprinter.

3. Quickly spring your foot off the ground instead of scraping it along the ground or pushing off with excessive force.

4. Don't overstride in front of you to go faster; this will wreck your knees and awkwardly stretch leg muscles.

5. Keep arms close to your side and relaxed with the elbows 90 degrees or less.

6. Don't swing your arms back and forth like you are a drum major in a marching band.

7. Hands should not be squeezed tight or balled in a fist, but relaxed and loosely cupped, thumbs gently grazing a finger or two.

8. Don't look at the ground right in front of your feet; look forward instead while trying to maintain relaxed facial muscles.

9. Don't run leaning too far forward.

10. Run upright or with slight forward lean from ankles, but not with your shoulders pulled back like a soldier at attention on the parade grounds.

— *Excerpted from* Return to Fitness: Getting Back in Shape After Injury, Illness, or Prolonged Inactivity, *by Bill Katovsky; and with assistance from Mark Cucuzzella, M.D.*

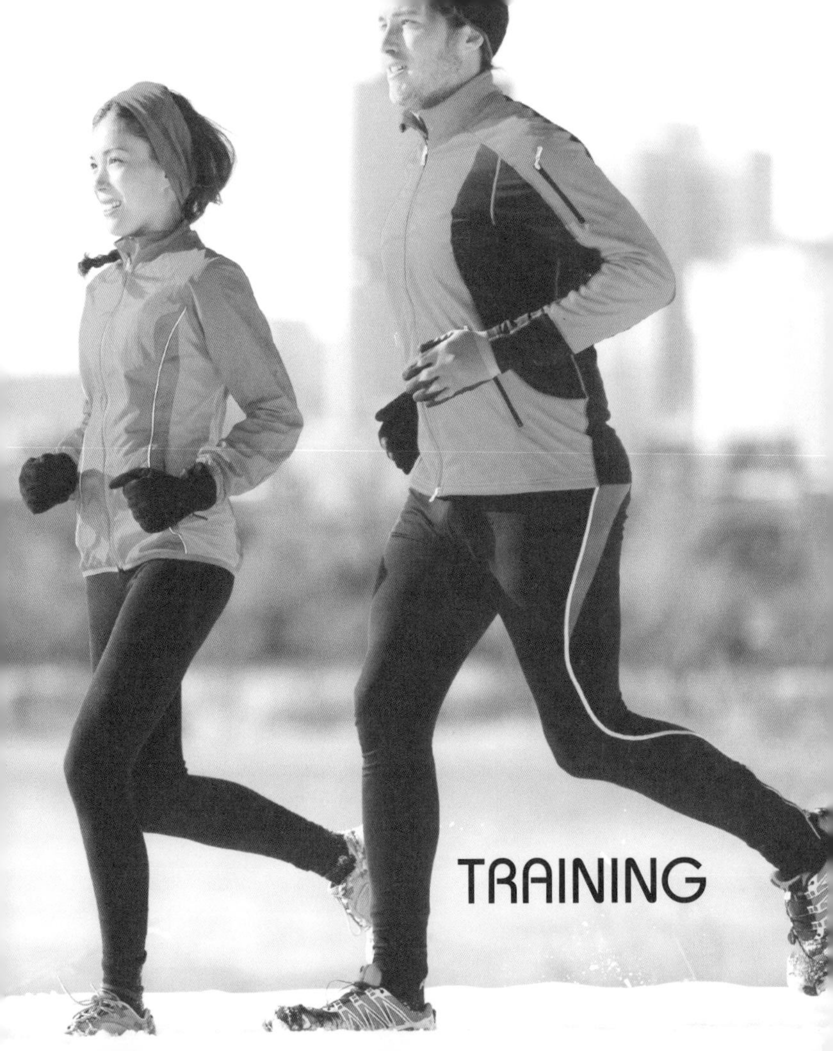

TRAINING

In one of his non-fiction bestsellers, Outliers, *Malcolm Gladwell introduces the idea that "practice makes perfect" is less of a cliché and more of a truism empirically based in reality. But how much* practice *does* perfection *actually demand? The number Gladwell arrives at is a staggering 10,000 hours if you want to become the very best in your field. This figure applies across all disciplines, including sports, business, music, chess, dance, art, science, and academics. Ten thousand hours is the dividing line between success and non-success, unquestioned excellence and muddling mediocrity.*

Of course, there's the underlying yet inescapable issue of natural talent. Only the fortunate few win the genetic jackpot by having the right set of parents. We cannot all aspire to be the next Mozart, Picasso, Michael Jordan, or one of the four Beatles. But does the 10,000 hour rule apply to runners? If you want to win the Olympic gold-medal in the marathon, will you need to log 10,000 hours of training? Can steely, unwavering determination trump innate ability or physical attributes that offer easily measured benefits such as VO2-max?

In 2000, the Danish Sports Science Institute conducted

a study of young Kenyan runners and theorized that their remarkable ability might be a result of their "birdlike legs." What the study failed to address is that Kenyans have a fierce work ethic when it comes to running. Early in the season, they will run three times a day. The elite marathoners will often run 150 miles per week in training. The Kenyans' commitment and love of running, which starts in childhood when they often run several miles a day to school, usually barefoot, serve as vivid and inspiring examples of what the human body is capable of achieving.

How about the rest of us? Let's say that at the impressionable age of 16, you start running an hour a day under the guidance of a strict, no-nonsense coach. By the end of year one, you would have trained 365 hours. And by the time you have finally banked those 10,000 hours, you will be 43 years old. That would make you six years older than the oldest Olympic marathon winner, Carlos Lopes, of Portugal, who took gold in the 1984 Los Angeles Olympics at the age of 37. At the Beijing Olympic Games, Constantina Dita Tomescu of Romania was 38 when she won the marathon.

If you can somehow double your workouts and make it to the 10,000 hour mark at a much earlier age, this still doesn't guarantee automatic Olympic success because the real point of Gladwell's thesis as it applies to running is not so much the actual number of hours one spends training, but the degree of one's commitment over a sustained period of time. In other words, if you want to get really good in this sport, whether you are a beginner or experienced age-grouper, you need to be smart and consistent with your training. You need to stay healthy and injury-free.

The average American takes twenty years to get out of condition and he wants to get back in condition in twenty days—and you just can't do it.

—Dr. Kenneth Cooper, author of 1968 best-seller *Aerobics*

Just as you write down other important appointments, you need to literally pencil in time for your run. The process itself is empowering. In the few seconds it takes to scribble "run" into a time slot, you make running a part of your life.

—Jeff Galloway

At my school, I was timekeeper. It was my responsibility to make sure the other students were on time. So it was important that I arrived always first.

—Ibraham Hussein, of Kenya and three-time winner of the Boston Marathon

There's a lot to be said for LSD—long, slow distance, in this case.

—Joe Henderson

I don't want to plead that it's the life of a monk, but I can't think of a sport—with the possible exception of swimming—where people train as hard.

—Sebastian Coe

The long run puts the tiger in the cat.

—Bill Squires, coach of the Greater Boston Track club at the height of its marathon success in the 70s and early 80s

Training = Workout + Rest

—Dr. Phil Maffetone, *The Big Book of Endurance Racing and Training*

In order to cash in on all the training, get the rest. If you can't run as fast as you want to, you haven't rested enough.
—Ted Corbitt, known as the "father of long-distance running" and U.S. National Marathon Champion in 1954

No one will burn out doing aerobic running. It is too much anaerobic running, which the American scholastic athletic system tends to put young athletes through, that burns them out.

—Arthur Lydiard

You can't burn the candle all the time. If you put in long miles as a teenager, how are you going to do it for twenty years after that?

—Bill Rodgers

My advice to young runners is to concentrate on track and cross-country. Take the gradual approach. Then, when you are in your twenties, experiment with longer road races. Just take a low-key approach. You can't tell in one year or two years what you are going to do.

—Bill Rodgers

I believe you'll develop speed via strength work, which includes hill running, or running hilly courses, as the Kenyans do on a steady basis.

—Bill Rodgers

Slow is the new fast.
—Bill Katovsky, author and editor loping along in his early 50s

Nothing gets in the way of my workout.

—Robert de Castella

The key ingredient, in my opinion, to successful mental training is what I refer to as a "warrior attitude."

—Bob Glover and Shelly-Lynn Florence Glover, *The Competitive Runner's Handbook*

On those mornings when I was tempted to roll over and fall asleep again, I imagined my racing rivals leaping out of bed and roaring out the front door on a ten-mile workout. The thought so terrified me that I was generally lacing up my shoelaces within five minutes.

—Amby Burfoot

I've been doing high mileage ever since day one. Mileage is nothing new to me. My legs respond better to it. For example, I've found that I can do really well for a 10K by putting in 120 miles a week. That's the kind of stuff I've been doing for my marathon training and that's when I feel my best. I've kind of found my niche.

—Ryan Hall, in 2008 interview in *California Track & Running News;* in 2011 at Boston, he ran the fastest marathon ever by an American, 2:04:58, finishing fourth

The introduction of resistance in form of sand and hill is too important to be ignored.

—Percy Cerutty, Australian running coach

A guy who has run twenty Boston Marathons was once asked, "Don't you feel like skipping a day when it's raining?" The old road warrior replied, "If you start skipping runs because the weather's too lousy, pretty soon you start missing runs because the weather's too nice!"

—Florence Griffith Joyner and Jon Hanc, *Running for Dummies*

The training is my secret and if I told you what it was, it wouldn't be a secret anymore! I keep the secret in my heart.

—Wilson Boit Kipketer, of Kenya and former world record-holder in the 3,000-meters steeplechase

Running is a number's game. You need to put in the training mileage. Just like making bank deposits before making a withdrawal

—Bill Katovsky

Runners like to train 100 miles per week because it's a round number. But I think 88 is a lot rounder.

—Don Kardong

Something that should lower stress can actually cause stress if it's done in the wrong spirit. Scientists put two rats in a cage, each of them locked inside a running wheel. The first rat could exercise whenever it liked. The second rat was forced to run whenever its counterpart did. Exercise, like meditation, usually tamps down stress and encourages neuron growth. The second rat, however, lost brain cells. It was doing something that should have been good for its brain, but it lacked one crucial factor: control. It could not determine its own "workout" schedule, so it didn't perceive it as exercise. Instead, it experienced it as a literal rat race.

—from 2009 *Newsweek* cover story, "Who Says Stress Is Bad For You?" by science reporter Mary Carmichael

Everyone is an athlete. The only difference is that some of us are in training, and some are not.

—George Sheehan, M.D.

What I did in those early months wasn't "training." It was more about trying not to get hurt than trying to get better.

—John Bingham

Frank [Shorter] had a rational judgment of what he could do. If he had a cold, or was busy in law school, he was always able to make a judgment not to kill himself and stay healthy.

—Kenny Moore

The ability to recover goes away as you age. What I've found is that my recovery is slower, and I can't do the pounding.

—Frank Shorter

In place of wasteful hobbies there commences a period of supervised and systematic physical training, together with instruction in the art of living fully. This replaces previously undirected life.

—Percy Cerutty

In my opinion, nothing beats a treadmill workout when you don't want to run outside. A good movie, some water, and a little ventilation are all you need.

—Florence Griffith Joyner

During the hard training phase, never be afraid to take a day off. If your legs are feeling unduly stiff and sore, rest; if you are at all sluggish, rest; in fact, if in doubt, rest.

—Bruce Fordyce, nine-time winner of the Comrades Marathon in South Africa

Train, don't strain.

—Arthur Lydiard

Most of my early training was experimental. I tested theories and techniques on myself. If they worked, I'd pass them on to my friends.

—Ted Corbitt

Does it work? Does it not? You learn by your mistakes. It's so subtle. If you run so hard that you can't recover, you haven't done any good.

—Roger Bannister

The most important day in any running program is rest. Rest days give your muscles time to recover so you can run again. Your muscles build in strength as you rest.

—Hal Higdon

I'll train like a madman, un loco. Well, not like a madman, perhaps, but as if it were my last race.

—Rodolfo Gomez, of Mexico, prior to the marathon at the Los Angeles Olympics

The will to win means nothing without the will to prepare.

—Juma Ikangaa, of Tanzania, second-place Boston Marathon finisher three consecutive years and two-time winner of Tokyo Marathon

If you talk to an elite or near-elite American distance runner today, they'll tell you that the primary aim of their training is to avoid injury. If you had talked to a similar athlete 25 years ago—somebody doing the '82 Boston, for example—he would have told you the idea of training was to run fast.

—Tom Derderian, coach of the Greater Boston Track Club

A lot of people think that they can "sweat out" a fever by running. They think that running will help their immune system fight it off. That's wrong.

—David Nieman, Ph.D., head of the Human Performance Laboratory, Appalachian State University

Hills are speedwork in disguise.

—Frank Shorter

Hills are the only beneficial type of resistance training for the runner.

—Arthur Lydiard

Say no to "no pain, no gain" and instead "train, don't strain."

—Bob Glover, *The Runner's Handbook*

Every runner has a perfect training level of weekly miles that will allow him or her to maximize performance and minimize injuries. Finding that level is not always easy to do.

—Hal Higdon

I looked at Paavo Nurmi and the rest of the great Finnish runners before the war, and I realized that what set them up, apart from the others of the day, was that they did high mileage.

—Arthur Lydiard

Once, it is said, he ran 40 miles from a small town to his home in Turku on the northwest coast of Finland. His wife heard a faint scratching on their back door. Thinking it was a neighborhood dog, she opened the door. There was Paavo [Nurmi], slumped in a heap on the doorstep, so exhausted from his run that he could not open the door.

—Michael Sandrock, *Running with the Legends;* Nurmi won five gold medals at the 1924 Olympics, including the 1,500 and 5,000 meters

Training is principally an act of faith. The athlete must believe in its efficacy; he must believe that through training he will become fitter and stronger; that by constant repetition of the same movements he will become more skillful and his muscles more relaxed.

—Franz Stampfl, *On Running*

Once upon a time, about twenty years ago to be precise, runners believed they didn't have to do anything but run.

—Amby Burfoot, *The Principles of Running*

What I was doing in the past was running my easy days too fast and not letting the body rest a bit, and then getting on the track and not putting in the times and the effort. And I was not fresh enough to enjoy what I was doing.

—Priscilla Welch

Everything I see and feel is more extreme when I'm in training. If I'm happy, I'm happier. If I'm sad, I'm sadder.

—Kathrine Switzer

It is amazing how much you can progress week after week, month after month, year after year if you allow for gradual training increases.

—Bob Glover, *The Runner's Handbook*

If you under-train, you may not finish, but if you over-train, you may not start.

—Stan Jensen, ultra-runner extraordinaire

My [early] training was very simple and very primitive.

—Emil Zatopek

When you're young and training two or three times a day, you can beat everybody your age, but you'll only last a few years.

—Arturo Barrios, of Mexico and former world-record holder of the 10,000 meters

I train for good luck.

—Arturo Barrios

Every so often, if you find your times slowing down, if you find your strength leaving you a little bit, don't try to push through it. Totally detrain.

—Priscilla Welch

You train best where you are the happiest.

—Frank Shorter

I noted in my diary four or five things I did wrong in preparation for the race: like needing more 25-30 mile training runs, doing more speedwork, and drinking more fluids during a race. Unfortunately, I forgot all that at the Olympics.

—Bill Rodgers on the 1976 Montreal Olympics

I train for good luck.

—Arturo Barrios

I have the mentality that I can train like a man, and it helps me a lot.

—Uta Pippig

Numbers don't lie. You always seem to remember your workouts as being a little better than they were. It's good to go back and review what you do.

—Frank Shorter

After 10 years of tough marathon training, it was time to give the body a rest. I really was tired, and I needed to recoup. I needed to go back to 60 to 70 miles per week.

—Priscilla Welch

Injuries made me a cross-training believer.

—Florence Griffith-Joyner

Pre[fontaine] was the hardest worker in running that I ever had by far. This is the whole thing, his intensity.

—Walt McClure

Success is the result of the application of scientific methods of training to the development of natural talents or skill, which we all possess in some degree or another.

—Walter George, late nineteenth century British runner whose world-record time for the mile (4:12) lasted for almost 30 years

Set aside a time solely for running. Running is more fun if you don't have to rush though it.

—Jim Fixx, author of 1977 bestseller *The Complete Book of Running*

I've learned that it's what you do with your miles, rather than how many you've run.

—Rod DeHaven, winner of U.S. 2000 Olympic Trials marathon (2:15:30)

What I would use [to run on the treadmill on the MIR space station] is bungee cords; it kind of looks like a windsurfer harness and that would yank me down with a spring force, if you will. It was the equivalent of loading your body up. It felt like carrying a heavy pack on your back. So it wasn't a natural run. It was not comfortable; plus you're just staring at walls inside of a cave. The only way I could get through those workouts was to close my eyes and literally visualize step-by-step a run that I would take on Earth. In the park, I could see the kids playing. I'd just escape the reality of where I was and just go back and use my imagination to get through the workout, and by doing that sometimes I'd find myself twenty-five minutes later virtually in front of my house. I'd finish my run and then I'd open my eyes and realize, of course, I'm in this space station. That's the way I was able to do the workouts.

—Jerry Linenger, NASA astronaut who spent 132 days aboard MIR

"Somewhere in the world someone is training when you are not. When you race him, he will win."

—Tom Fleming, winner of the 1973 and 1975 New York City Marathon, and two time *runner*-up in the Boston Marathon

The day I walk into the home of any runner in any African city, town, or village and find a StairMaster, rowing machine, or wet vest near a swimming pool, I'll be proved wrong. Until that day, I stick by my belief in the need to concentrate on putting in the running miles.

—Tom Fleming

I'd run from my house down two blocks and back and lie on the ground and die.

—Jim Ryun on training when he was fifteen

People sometimes say runners like my father and other Kenyan runners win because they are talented. There's no secret. All there is is hard work, just training very hard. That's how my father did it, and that's how the others are doing it.

—Martin Keino, son of Kenyan running great Kipchoge Keino, and the 1994 NCAA cross country and 1995 NCAA 5,000-meters champion

I've had only one utterly dependable training partner: a golden retriever named Rockee. We were joined at the hip for fourteen years and 7,000 miles of running together. Rockee was a sixty-five-pound bundle of crazy canine love, with a white clown face that turned even whiter as he got older. He never once complained if we ran too far, or if I were going too slow. I never heard him go on and on about an injury, like so many runners do. He never bellyached if the weather was too hot or too cold. He just loved to run, especially on the trails. His limitless energy and unflagging enthusiasm were inspiring to behold. He got me running on those days when I was tempted to find an excuse not to put on my Asics or Nikes, slip on the sweat bandana, grab his red leash, and head outside. Memories are man's best friend.

—Bill Katovsky

The purpose of training is to stress the body, so when you rest it will grow stronger and more tolerant of the demands of distant running.

—*David Costill,* professor of exercise science at Ball State University

I leave my watch at home. Otherwise, it's a lost cause.

—Todd Williams, two-time U.S. cross-country champion (1991 and 1992), on what he must do to have an easy workout

I find 140 miles per week is easy, but 160 is hard.

—Tom Fleming, in 1979, while training for the Boston Marathon

It is a belief that finds no support in other fields of endeavor. The child learning to write, the pianist who practices for six hours a day, the bricklayer laying bricks—the work of these people does not deteriorate as a result of constant repetition of the same movements.

—Franz Stampfl

Did the cat do stretches? Did the cat jog around? Did the cat do knee bends? Did the cat have a track suit on before racing? No, the cat just got up and went. No more warming up. Forget it.

—Percy Cerutty, to his team after dumping a bucket of water on a cat and watching it run away

Why should I practice running slow? I already know how to run slow. I want to learn to run fast. Everyone said: 'Emil, you are a fool!' But when I first won the European Championship, they said: 'Emil, you are a genius!'"

—Emil Zatopek, concerning his emphasis on interval training

I had over-trained. I put too much pressure on myself because I wanted that gold medal too much. If I had trained 15 percent less, I would have won. I was training like a crazy person. There was a lack of self-confidence and a lack of maturity. An athlete does not only train with his body. He trains with his mind.

—Hicham El Guerrouj, of Morocco, on his second-place finish in the 1,500 meters at the 2000 Olympics

When you're running 190 miles a week, you do nothing else. You have to live like a monk.

—Pablo Sierra, winner of 1994 Twin Cities Marathon

Overtraining is the biggest problem incurred by runners who lack the experience or discipline to cope with their own enthusiasm.

—Marty Liquori

If someone says, "Hey I ran 100 miles this week. How far did you run?" ignore him! What the hell difference does it make? The magic is in the man, not the 100 miles.

—Bill Bowerman

There is no path I follow. I feel as if I'm just drifting along, because although I can progress physically, through my training, mentally and spiritually I don't know what the hell I'm doing. It's like that car sticker: "Don't follow me, I'm lost."

—Steve Ovett, British gold medalist in the 800 meters at the 1980 Olympics, and former world record holder in the 1,500 meters and mile (3:48)

I use my running (and deliberately shun the word "training") as the daily reset button. The harder and busier the day is the more I need to do an easy run. This relaxation counters the sometime toxic levels of stress that comes with being overextended as a family physician and other work commitments. If running were another stress it would not be sustainable, therefore all of my running is relaxed. Often people read schedules developed by elite athletes and they have weekly strenuous sessions. Now if you are an elite athlete and the rest of your day is the relaxing part then you can add frequent stressful workouts. For 99.9 percent of all runners this is not the case. We all have busy and stressful lives and the running must fit into the "yin" of the "yin and yang" circle.

—Mark Cucuzzella, M.D.

Ten Smart Training Tips *from* The Little Red Book of Running, *by Scott Douglas (Skyhorse Publishing)*

There Are No Junk Miles

If you're not injured so badly that you're altering your form, or so sick that you feel much worse after running, then it's all good. Even if you think a run doesn't advance your fitness, it has other benefits—promoting blood flow, clearing your mind, getting you away from the computer, burning calories, getting you out in nature, helping you spend time with friends, giving you much-needed time by yourself, maintaining the rhythm of good training, and infinitely so on.

Always Let the Pace Come to You

Even if you're not trying to run more, start out a lot slower than you'll be running when you finish. Easing into runs and gradually picking up the pace as feels comfortable is one of the keys to making more runs enjoyable and fruitful.

We're All Slower Than Somebody

There's nothing to be gained from belittling yourself over how fast you can run; banish all thoughts of, "Oh, I'm so slow, what's the point?" People get lapped even in world-class 10Ks on the track.

Keep Gadgets in Their Place

Too many runners over-rely on their measuring gadgets during normal runs, when it's not important to hit specific combinations of time and distance. To them, a run is successful only if the gadget spits out the right numbers. It's worth making this point again: A mile has no meaning to the human body. You're imposing artificial definitions of success on your running by letting a device that speaks only in those measurements tell you if you had a good run.

Some Days, Leave the Watch at Home

At least a few days a week, decide what course you're going to run, and then leave your watch at home. Other days, run wherever, guided by total time on your watch. The thing to mostly avoid is timing yourself over the same courses day after day. In that way lies the madness of beating yourself up for running slower than you "should" or forcing yourself to pick it up because you're 6 seconds slower at your 45-minutes-into-it checkpoint than you were yesterday.

Love the Long Run

Doing one run a week that's significantly longer than most of your other runs is a great way to simultaneously boost your mileage and your fitness. Your main motivation for regularly doing long runs should be the latter—building your endurance so that all of your runs become more manageable. But I'm not going to deny that starting the week with a long run is a killer kick-off to meeting your weekly mileage goal. Near-weekly long runs are, of course, one of the backbones of marathon-training plans. Almost all runners looking to race well from 5K on up know the value of the long run.

Hit the Hills

More runners should do hard workouts on hills more regularly. Running hard uphill gives you all the benefits of running hard on flat ground, and then some—greater running-specific leg strength, more muscle fibers recruited (and therefore given an inducement to adapt to a higher work capacity), and, of course, specific preparation for tackling hills in races. Runners who might be a little insecure and in need of constant data-driven feedback on their fitness tend to shy away from hill workouts. And that's a shame, because there are several types of hill workouts that are highly effective at making you faster.

Short Hills

Fairly steep hills that take you between 30 and 60 seconds to get up are a staple of Kenyans' training.

Medium Hills

Hills that take about 90 seconds to climb are great for running economy workouts. If, however, you get to the bottom and aren't yet ready to go hard again, jog around a bit more. Hitting the proper intensity is much more important than simply being out of breath the whole time.

Long Hills

Hills that take two to four minutes to climb can serve many of the purposes of VO_2 max workouts.

"HEY COACH!"

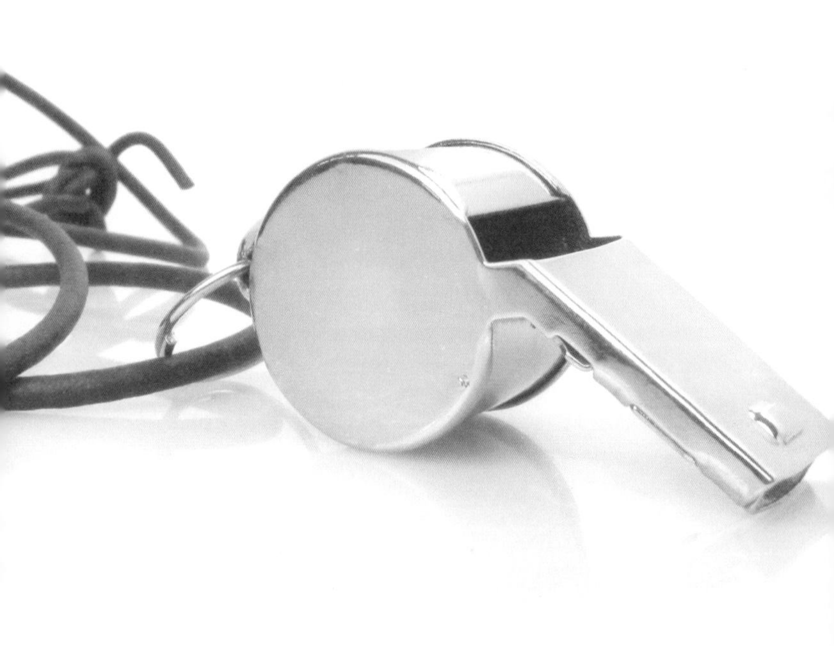

Past high school and college, it was usually only the top competitive runners who had the privilege or opportunity to work with a personal coach. Now recreational runners everywhere can easily find coaches that meet their athletic needs and interests. This recent phenomenon is a result of several factors: the relentless popularity of half-marathon and marathon charity races and organizations like Team in Training; an army of coaches and personal trainers offering their services online; and specialty running stores regularly holding clinics. Getting a coach or gait expert to assist your running or create a workout plan is a lot simpler these days.

Celebrities now rely on coaches for marathon training. One of the first, Oprah contacted Telluride Ski Resort head fitness instructor Bob Greene in the spring of 1993. The afternoon talk show host had a vacation home in the Colorado town and had gone on several hikes with Greene. She weighed 222 pounds, yet was determined to achieve "healthy weight loss." Under his dietary and training guidance, her early workout sessions involved a mix of jogging and walking – but only several miles. She averaged about 17 minutes per mile. By mid-summer, the weight was melting off Oprah's body as she increased her weekly mileage and pace. She was running five miles a day at a 10 to 11 minute-per-mile clip. Greene entered her in the San Diego half-marathon, and a 2:16 finish gave Oprah the confidence to train for the full marathon the following year. Greene defensively told the media at the time, "Sometimes people will say to me, 'Oprah's got it easy because she has a personal chef and a personal trainer.' But that's baloney. No one can run for you. She was on the track every morning. She worked herself as hard as any athlete I've seen. She deserved the results she achieved."

With weekly mileage approaching 50 miles, she was adequately prepared for the Marine Corps Marathon in the fall. A slim, fit, energized, and exuberant Oprah clocked 4:29 in the race; she didn't walk a step. "She's a runner now for life," her proud coach told reporters. (Most unfortunately, she later stopped running when the intense pressures of work and personal issues once again took over her life; in the past several years, she regained all the lost weight and more.) When Olympic speed-skating sprint champion Apolo Ohno decided to do a marathon, he used a coach to whip his muscular body into leaner long-distance running shape. He completed the 2011 New York City marathon in a respectable

3:24:14. As the winningest U.S. winter Olympian in history with a tally of eight medals, Ohno has a fierce work ethic when it came to training, but even his run coach and trainer Todd Rushworth needed to flex his mentoring chops during their workouts together. "I had to remind [Apolo] these were just training runs," he told Sports Illustrated. *"This is not your day. The hardest thing was getting him to slow down. And to eat."*

Now, let's hear from some of the coaching greats.

Only think of two things—the gun and the tape. When you hear the one, just run like hell until you break the other.

—Early 1900s British track coach Sam Mussabini, whose runners won a total of eleven medals over five Olympics; he was portrayed by actor Ian Holm in *Chariots of Fire*

Coaching an elite runner is something like driving an expensive car. The coach's main job is to steer.

—John Babington, longtime coach of the Wellesley College cross country and track team

If a man coaches himself, then he has only himself to blame when he is beaten.

—Roger Bannister

A coach can be like an oasis in the desert of a runner's lost enthusiasm.

—Ken Doherty, American decathlon champion in the late 1920s, author *of the Track & Field Omnibook,* and long-time college track coach (Michigan, Princeton, and University of Pennsylvania)

I tell my athletes, "When you compete, concentrate on yourself. Don't focus on anger against a competitor."

—Joe Douglas, founder of the Santa Monica Track Club whose athletes (including Carl Lewis) have won 27 Olympic medals and set 60 American records.

Different people come with different talents, but all runners need to be aerobic and able to supply oxygen at a certain tempo for a long period of time and have lactic acid tolerance.

—Joe Douglas

Weight training doesn't help runners move faster. But it can prevent injuries and it's motivational. That's why I use it.

—Joe Douglas

Runners should do a little work on their abdominals, because it helps keep their body mechanics comfortable. Training biceps and triceps doesn't do anything in running. If you were running on your hands it might be good, but you're not.

—Joe Douglas

I've had athletes say, "Boy, he's a strong runner." And I look at them because I honestly don't know what they're talking about. Does it mean he won the race? Does it mean he takes long steps? Does it mean he has a big chest? Does it mean he can go for a long time? Does it mean it's anaerobic? Aerobic? What does it mean? I don't know.

—Joe Douglas

You run the race, not the coach.

—Joe Douglas

You can't flirt with the track. You must marry it.

—Bill Easton, legendary coach at Drake and University of Kansas, and whose teams won six NCCA titles

The coach's main job is 20 percent technical and 80 percent inspirational.

—Franz Stampfl who helped train Roger Bannister before becoming a top Australian track coach; he helped pioneer interval training

A teacher is never too smart to learn from his pupils. But while runners differ, basic principles never change. So it's a matter of fitting your current practices to fit the event and the individual. See, what's good for you might not be worth a darn for the next guy.

—Bill Bowerman, co-founder of Nike, trained 24 NCAA champions and 16 sub-four-minute milers during his 24 years as coach at the University of Oregon

Bill Bowerman was, and is, and ever shall be a generous, ornery, profane, beatific, unyielding, antic, impenetrably complex Oregon original.

—Kenny Moore, who ran at University of Oregon, and set the U.S. marathon record (2:13:29) in 1969

I do give the athletes a relatively free rein and for good reason. One of my principles is, "Don't overcoach."

—Bill Bowerman

God determines how fast you're going to run; I can help only with the mechanics.

—Bill Bowerman

I do think there are lots of kids out there who have the potential to be great runners if only they have the right coach—someone who shows an interest and cares.

—Bill Rodgers

Coaching is no different from what a choreographer does with a dance or what a playwright does with a play.

—Brooks Johnson, Stanford University track and running coach

I've been running for over 20 years; I read all the books and articles, yet I need a coach. Why? I still have to be told, to be encouraged.

—Fred Lebow

I have a few requirements about who I will coach. I think a person has to stay with a program at least one year. That's the only way to know if it works. If I sense an athlete won't stick with a program, I won't work with him or her.

—Tom Fleming

The ability to make a man go beyond the point at which he thinks he is going to die.

—Franz Stampfl on what coaches need

Live like a clock.

—Jumbo Elliott, long-time Villanova track coach, on how runners should structure their lifestyle

Act like a horse. Be dumb. Just run.

—Jumbo Elliott

[Jumbo Elliott] forever sought "the wolf," the anchorman, the one who would make up the distance to the runner up ahead. His runners overachieved at times, became wolves to avoid disappointment in them—or to avoid his occasional outbursts.

—Theodore J. Berry, M. D., in *Jumbo Elliott: Makers of Milers, Maker of Men*

Most people need a coach to tell them to work hard; I need a coach to tell me to ease up.

—Marty Liquori, in 1975, ran a personal best 3:52.2 in the mile

I get more gratification out of getting some obese person who had a heart attack running around and enjoying life within a year. I get more gratification from that than putting a person in the Olympic games.

—Arthur Lydiard, legendary New Zealand coach and father of Long Slow Distance (LSD) and "jogging"

There is nothing more monotonous and *sickening* than running round and round a track.

—Arthur Lydiard on his aversion to pure interval training

Well, no athlete respects a big, fat coach who's going to stand there and rest the watch on his stomach.

—Arthur Lydiard

Don't attack a hill from the very bottom—it's bigger than you are!

—Harry Groves, Penn State coach

Everybody and their mother knows you don't train hard on Friday, the day before a race. But a lot of runners will overtrain on Thursday if left on their own. Thursday is the most dangerous day of the week.

—Marty Stern, Villanova women's coach and six-time NCAA "National Coach of the Year"

Coaching is an art and I'm not going to let anyone change me.

—Marty Stern

One of my biggest desires as a coach is to help adults learn to run like they did as kids. It's such a natural movement when kids do it.

—George Xu, T'ai Chi master

Ten years ago when I started coaching (at Cal State San Marcos) I stopped identifying myself as an athlete. I stopped identifying myself as the American record-holder. So the time I started coaching, I was a coach and all that matters to me was my coaching and my athletes and the old mile-record was just something that was nice.

—Steve Scott, who ran 136 sub-4-minute miles during his storied career

It's so gratifying to take a kid—recruiting them, bringing them in, working with them, developing them and then having them achieve their goals, even if their goals are far below what I achieved or other people are achieving at other universities. When you help them through that whole process and they improve and are happy with their performance, as a coach it can't make me any happier.

—Steve Scott, in 2008 *Running Times* interview

"Bill Squires was the Best Marathon Coach in U.S. History"

— Bill Rodgers

Bill Squires coached the Greater Boston Track club (Bill Rodgers, Alberto Salazar, Dick Beardsley and Greg Meyer) at the height of its marathon success in the 1970s and early 1980s; the following quotes are from a 2011 Running Times interview profile by Scott Douglas

My athletes, I never pushed them on distance. If they started going on the loopy stuff, 125, 160 miles a week, I said, 'Go with Rodgers. He has to do that.' He must love seeing the birds and squirrels and all that crap.

—Bill Squires

We start talking workouts, and he wants to show me his training log. I said, "Jesus Christ, I don't wanna read that thing. The only thing I read is the obituaries in the morning paper to see if I'm still alive."

— Bill Squires, on coaching Dick Beardsley

Running is a simple sport. You don't need all the zoopy zoopy.

—Bill Squires

[Alberto Salazar as a teen] looked like a broken down old man. If he hadn't come to me before college, he would have never gotten into Oregon. He was a very bright kid—I thought he was going to go to med school. I would have chosen not one of my athletes if I was recruiting for a Division I school.

—Bill Squires

I had to pull [Bill Rodgers] aside and give him the facts of life. I said, "Look pal, we're just little nerds who are kicking the world around. None of you people would I pick to be outstanding. But the program works. If you want to radio it out to the world they're going to kick your can, because they're better than you, ya hear me? You're only good with the group I trained. So just shut your mouth!"

—Bill Squires

I'm not into these practice runners, the Cinderfellas, who want a Purple Heart for their workout. I always say, Let's see what we do on Saturday [in the race].

—Bill Squires

One thing I took away from Squires is that there's a lot of different ways to get fit. I don't remember Squires ever talking about times in the marathon. He only talked about strategy and beating people. If you get people to believe and if they're happy, they tend to do well.

—Greg Meyer, last American to win the Boston Marathon race (1983), in 2:09.

I totally believed everything he told me. If he had told me to go sit in a garbage can, I'd have done it.

—Dick Beardsley, on Bill Squires

I learned quickly that if I had to talk to Coach on the phone, I'd better do it early in the day. If I talked to him at, say, eight o'clock at night, I couldn't get to sleep. I wanted to run the workout right then. He'd get me so fired up I'd just lie in bed feeling the adrenaline pound its way through my body.

—Dick Beardsley, on Bill Squires

I have a thing with exercise physiologists. They only work with established runners. They can't coach a cat to meow. To be a marathon coach, you better run the marathon. You don't have to be a speed demon but you have to do it.

—Bill Squires, who ran a 2:47 in the 1961 Boston Marathon and finished in 20th place

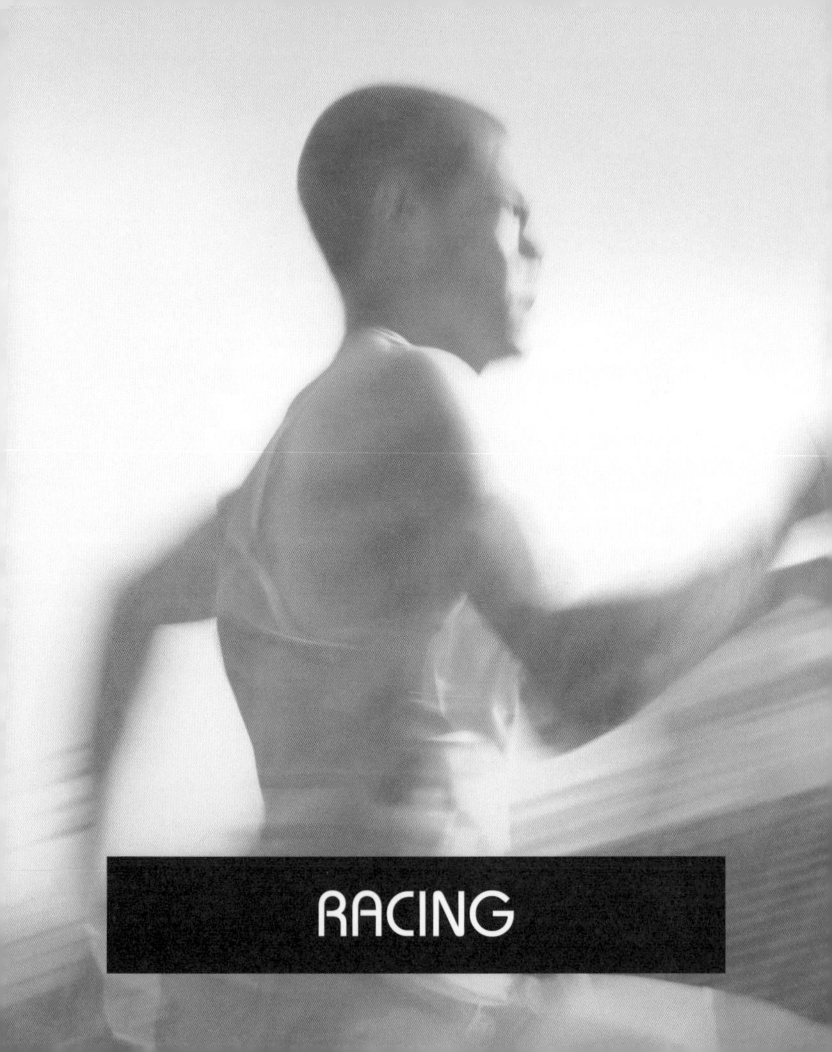
RACING

When I was twenty-two, I took up running for the first time, in part to emotionally recuperate from college love gone sour. This was 1979. The summer before, I biked solo across America. Running seemed like a good addition to my athletic resume. I'd occasionally run several miles and found that the longer I ran, the better I felt. At the time, running and cycling lived in fenced-off athletic ghettos. But by combining biking and running, I never got injured. My knees held up fine, always a concern for runners. I was running between ten and fifteen miles a week in beat-up Adidas tennis sneakers.

In October 1981, I impulsively entered my first running race, a 13.1-mile hilly affair in Berkeley, California, where I now lived and toiled in the academic salt mines as a political science graduate student. I hadn't trained specifically for this race. Earlier that week, I had come across a flyer for the Berkeley-to-Moraga half-marathon in a bookstore on Telegraph Avenue. I was curious about running that far. The farthest I had ever run was 10 miles in a single stretch and that had been over a year ago. Since I didn't run with a watch, I didn't care a whit about a predicted time, or even knew what it meant.

When I showed up on that cold fall morning near the

entrance to the grand Claremont Hotel, there were about two hundred runners already gathered on a side street, many hopping about in order to stay warm. Almost everyone seemed to know one another. I noticed several guys wearing red or blue running tights. I had never seen that before. I thought runners only wore shorts.

I seeded myself in the back and waited for the race to begin. The first 4.5 miles went straight uphill, first along a steep section of Ashby Avenue and then the switch-backing Tunnel Road, where all the homes would go up in smoke ten years later in the devastating Oakland fire. I started out too fast and struggled in oxygen-debt, but I edged back, recovered my wind, and paced myself on the gradual climb. I must have been in the top half of the field at the 1,200-foot summit, feeling cocky and smug at my unexpected success; but on the subsequent two-mile flat section, runner after runner zipped right past me. My legs felt leaden and unresponsive.

The course descended into a heavily forested canyon for several miles. Near the eight- or nine-mile mark, I asked a runner who had pulled aside me, "How are you feeling? Tired?" My legs had the consistency of concrete.

"No," she replied. "I feel fine."

"I'm curious, but can you tell me how much training you do?"

"About thirty or forty miles a week," she replied, before peeling away. There was no way I could keep up with her.

Running is a numbers game, I thought. You need to put in the training mileage to do well in a race. I grinded out the remaining miles, finishing the race in a mental and physical fog of 1:45, or just over eight minutes per mile. I received a small, yellow fabric finisher's patch. I never checked the final standings to see where I placed, though someone had posted the top ten times—all in the 70-minute range. The following day, I came down with the flu and spent the next 72 hours shaking and shivering in bed because I had overstressed my immune system. My body paid the penalty for being undertrained for a race of this toughness.

Many people new to running first decide to compete in a race like the half-marathon or full marathon, and only then do they begin the disciplined regimen of training. It's the current modus operandi *for countless charity-run participants and first-timers whose lives now happily revolve around this healthy, transformative obsession. Training schedules are carefully mapped out and workouts proudly logged to achieve maximum results in the shortest amount of time.*

While it's entirely possible to finish a marathon within six months of training, many coaches recommend several years of serious training. In the end, there's no right way or wrong way to train for a race, so long as you enjoy running. Distance is finite; speed is relative.

This chapter covers the gamut of racers and racing, from front-runners to back-of-the-packers and everyone else in-between.

When you cross the finish line, no matter how slow or fast, it will change your life forever.

—from *Spirit of the Marathon*, a documentary focusing on several runners in the Chicago Marathon

A lot of people run a race to see who's the fastest. I run to see who has the most guts.

—Steve Prefontaine

I have been passed in races by tall runners and short runners. I have been passed by runner who look as though they have not eaten in six weeks, and by runners who appear to have just wiped out an all-you-can-eat breakfast bar.

—John Bingham, author of *The Courage to Start*

Why run a race? You race to test yourself, for the ritual, the camaraderie, and for the adventure and discovery.

—from *The New York Road Runners Club Complete Book of Running*

My times become slower and slower, but the experience of the race is unchanged: each race a drama, each race a challenge, each race stretching me in one way or another, and each race telling me more about myself and others.

—George Sheehan, M.D.

Running is the ultimate tortoise-and-hare activity because the tortoise wins all of the important races. Oh, sure, the hare might get a gold medal at the Olympics or Boston Marathon. But it's the tortoises who continue to run for decades and often even for a lifetime.

—Amby Burfoot, author of *The Principles of Running*

As runners, we all go through many transitions—transitions that closely mimic the larger changes we experience in a lifetime. First, we try to run faster. Then we try to run harder. Then we learn to accept ourselves and our limitations, and at last, we can appreciate the true joy and meaning of running.

—Amby Burfoot

In many ways, a race is analogous to life itself. Once it is over, it can not be re-created. All that is left are impressions in the heart, and in the mind.

—Chris Lear, author of *Running with the Buffaloes*

He was the first to transform the 5,000 and 10,000 into a protracted sprint. That is how he felt he was his best. Because before Lasse, nobody ever went that early.

—Frank Shorter on how Lasse Viren, four-time Olympic gold medalist, changed racing tactics

He put his elbows on his knees and just slowly looked around at everyone in the room, one by one, as if to say, "I'm here, guys." And the race was over then. I've never seen a presence like that.

—Garry Bjorklund, on Viren before the 1976 Montreal Olympics

In Finland, we have a saying, "Big words don't fell the trees." That's what Lasse did in his running. His races speak louder than his words.

—Eino Romppanen, Finnish runner and sculptor

An athlete's career is a brief lightning flash; let me do as much as I can with it before it ends.

—Lasse Viren

When I see a videotape of the race, I think of how much fun it would have been to attend as a spectator . . . just to watch. Let alone be in it. Even watching a tape today, it makes the hair on the back of my neck stand up.

—Dick Beardsley, on losing by two seconds in the 1982 Boston Marathon "Duel in the Sun" with Alberto Salazar

Beardsley: "You ran a hell of a race."
Salazar: "You had me hurting."

—Exchange between both just past the Boston finish line

Sooner or later, someone always asks about the '82 Boston. I don't mind—I like talking about it, and so does Dick. That's because we never discuss the race in terms of running a 2:08 or beating the other guy. It took us both a long, long time, but we finally realized that that's not what the marathon is really about.

—Alberto Salazar

I think it comes down to pride in the end. Not proud, necessarily, that you're better than everybody else, but that you are tougher than anybody else. That if you lose, you are going to make whomever you are running against pay.

—Alberto Salazar

I felt decent immediately after [the 1982 Boston Marathon], but started to feel faint at the awards ceremony. I went to the underground garage where they gave me fluids. Have you ever had a cramp in your foot? It felt like I had a cramp in my entire body. In retrospect, I surely didn't drink enough during the race. I took no water at all over the last eight miles. I've never said this before, but I feel that one race had a lot to do with my health problems in later years. I feel I permanently damaged my thermoregulatory system on that day. Although I went on to run well on the track that summer, I never was the same and it all went downhill after that. If asked whether it was worth it, I would have to say yes. It means a great deal to have won that race.

—Alberto Salazar, in an interview with Don Allison of CoolRunning.com

I'd rather run a gutsy race, pushing all the way and lose, than run a conservative race only for a win.

—Alberto Salazar

No athlete was ever tougher than Joan Benoit, and no one more defining in her cycle of injury, recovery, victory, and injury—of love and loving too much.

—Kenny Moore, on Joan Benoit Samuelson

When you are really successful you have an aura about you that makes opponents not only a little bit wary of you, but makes them a little bit afraid of you, and consider you a threat.

—Frank Shorter

We were two individuals who both wanted to be the best in the U.S., and being the best in the U.S. at that time pretty much meant you were the best in the world.

—Frank Shorter, on he and Bill Rodgers

It's something in me, deep down, that makes me different in a race.

—Eamon Coghlin

You know, fourth is the absolutely worst place to finish in the Olympics.

—Eamonn Coghlan

People claim that fourth is the worst place to finish in the Olympics or Olympic Trials. Maybe, but I finished fifth in one Olympic Trials, and I much rather would have finished fourth.

—Hal Higdon

When I crossed the finish line in first place at the World Masters Championships in Finland, I knelt and kissed the track. It embarrassed my wife sitting in the stands, but it was the track that had carried me to victory.

—Hal Higdon

He ran like a "green" three-year-old thoroughbred having its first race in a classic—running all over the track, on the inside, then the outside, accelerating and slowing up before making his final effort, to finish fourth.

—*The Daily Mirror* on Roger Bannister's failure at the 1952 Helsinki Olympics

One thing about racing is that it hurts. You better accept that from the beginning or you're not going anywhere.

—Bob Kennedy, U.S. 5,000-meters record holder and first non-African under 13 minutes

Stupid, blind determination forced me on.

—Peter Snell, of New Zealand, and three-time Olympic gold medalist (800 meters and 1,500 meters)

Finishing that 5K was the hardest thing I ever had to do. I ate more fettuccine Alfredo, and drank less water than I have in my entire life. People always talk about triumphs of the human spirit. Today I had a triumph of the human body. My guts. My heart. While I eventually puked my guts out, I never puked my heart out. And I am very, very proud of that.

—Michael, from *The Office*

Marathons are extraordinarily difficult, but if you've got the training under your belt, and if you can run smart, the races take care of themselves.

—Deena Kastor, first American women to run a sub-2:20 marathon

As athletes, we have ups and downs. Unfortunately, you can't pick the days they come on.

—Deena Kastor on fracturing her foot shortly after the marathon start at the Beijing Olympic Games

To avoid starting out too fast, you have to "have eyes in your stomach." As we say in Norwegian, "a good gut instinct of control."

—Grete Waitz

Sex before the race? Fine, it will do you no harm. But try not to distract the starter.

—Roger Robinson, author, masters runner

I went at each race like there was a gold medal at stake. It wasn't like I ran one hard, then slacked off the next. Every time it was my best effort. I didn't know how to go at it any other way.

—Dick Beardsley

Every time he beat me I became more resolved. I would test him and could never find a flaw. He was a real, real student of the sport.

—Garry Bjorklund, top record-setting collegiate runner, on Bill Rodgers

I compare it to a kid having a big jar of candy. At the beginning, you're stuffing your face with candy. Then, when you have only about a half-dozen pieces left, you start to savor them. You treat every race like it's special.

—Marcus O'Sullivan, of Ireland and three-time world indoor champion in the 1,500 meters, on the end of his racing career

I have to give up so many things, make so many personal sacrifices, to perform at my level, that I cannot even contemplate losing.

—Sebastian Coe, two-time Olympic gold medalist in the 1,500 meters

The great thing about athletics is that it's like poker sometimes: you know what's in your hand and it may be a load of rubbish, but you've got to keep up the front.

—Sebastian Coe

The possibilities in racing tactics are almost unlimited, as in a game of chess, for every move there is a counter, for every attack there is a defense.

—Franz Stampfl, *Franz Stampfl on Running*

There is something about the ritual of the race—putting on the number, lining up, being timed—that brings out the best in us.

—Grete Waitz

I pray.

—Meb Keflezighi, who won the 2012 U.S. Olympic Marathon Trial, when asked what he does in a race when the going gets tough

The Australian behavior toward losers is far from healthy. If youngsters are taught that losing is a disgrace, and if they're not sure they can win, they will be reluctant to even try. And not trying is the real disgrace.

—Ron Clarke

When you put yourself on the line in a race and expose yourself to the unknown, you learn things about yourself that are very exciting

—Doris Brown Heritage, pioneer in women's distance running and winner of the world cross-country championships from 1967 to 1972

A road race is the closest thing to a party I can think of.

—from *Bill Rodgers' Lifetime Running Plan*

I love controlling a race, chewing up an opponent. Let's get down and dirty. Let's fight it out. It's raw, animalistic, with no one to rely on but yourself. There's no better feeling than that.

—Adam Goucher, winner of 1999 U.S. Nationals 5,000 meters

While a man is racing he must hate himself and his competitors.

—Percy Cerutty

A race is a work of art that people can look at and be affected by in as many ways as they're capable of understanding.

—Steve Prefontaine

I train to race. I love to train, but I love to race even more.

—Lynn Jennings

A slight hesitance, a single step to the inside, a few seconds miscalculation of the right pace of the timing of the final kick, and any other seemingly minor error, may throw away months and years of careful preparation and sacrifice.

—Ken Doherty, 1928 American decathlon champion

Often I visualize a quicker, almost like a ghost runner, ahead of me with a quicker stride. It's really crazy. In races, this always happens to me.

—Gabe Jennings

The most challenging aspect of the decathlon is not the events themselves, but how you train to become the best 100-meters runner you are on the same day that you're the best 1,500-meters runner.

—Bruce Jenner, winner of the 1976 Olympic decathlon

One of the things that made [Bill Rodgers] so great was his ability to lock down and focus for months at a time. Then during the race itself, he was just a freak, with incredible concentration. It goes back to that single-mindedness. When Billy charts a path, it's hard to get him to deviate from it.

—Greg Meyer

In any running event, you are absolutely alone. Nobody can help you.

—John Landy, of Australia, the second person to break four minutes in the mile

Kip [Keino] had what the best runners all have—the instinct to psych out your opponents in whatever way you can.

—Frank Shorter

His front-running example reinforced in my mind that that was the way you showed what you were made of—lead from the front, not just wait in the back.

—Alberto Salazar, on Steve Prefontaine

The minute Pre[fontainte] hit the field for his jog, there was an undercurrent of enthusiasm in the crowd. It surfaced in slight cheers as he raced down the stretch. You could feel the electricity.

—Geoff Hollister, University of Oregon runner and one of Nike's first employees

Racing is the reward your give yourself from all the hard training you put in, but can it lead to injury or burnout? Yes!

—Dick Beardsley

Without a race every so often, I lose the sense of awe at what I can do when I press myself, and at the same time I know my humility. I forget that racing can make the impossible possible and the possible impossible. Only here can I end up running faster than I ever thought I could or unable to cover a distance I've gone a thousand times before. Every race is a question, and I will never know until the last yards what the answer will be. That's the lure of racing.

—Joe Henderson, *The Long Run Solution*

Billy was a little intimidating when he was racing. He was a nice guy, except when he was racing. In a race, he became an animal and would do anything to beat you.

—Benji Durden, ranked among the top ten U.S. marathoners for six consecutive years, on Bill Rodgers

The start of a World Cross Country event is like riding a horse in the middle of a buffalo stampede. It's a thrill if you keep up, but one slip and you're nothing but hoof prints.

—Ed Eyestone

Get out well, but not too quickly, move through the field, be comfortable. Strategy-wise, go with your strengths. If you don't have a great finish, you must get away to win. I've always found it effective to make a move just before the crest of a hill. You get away just a little and you're gone before your opponent gets over the top. Also, around a tight bend, take off like holy hell. I've done that a number of times. You should not be flying down the home straight. Most of your efforts should have been put forth earlier.

—John Treacy, Ireland's two-time world cross country champion (1978, 1979)

Jogging through the forest is pleasant, as is relaxing by the fire with a glass of gentle Bordeaux and discussing one's travels. Racing is another matter. The frontrunner's mind is filled with an anguished fearfulness, a panic, which drives into pain.

—Kenny Moore

No one knows the fear in a frontrunner's mind more than me. When you set off at a cracking pace for four or five laps and find that your main rivals are still breathing down your neck, that's when you start to panic.

—Ron Clarke

As I stepped onto the track I felt my legs go rubbery. I saw over a 100,000 people in the stands, and before I knew it, I had collapsed onto the infield grass. "Can it be," I remembered thinking, as I lay there gazing up at the sky, "that I'm so nervous I'm not going to be able to run?" Then I realized how ridiculous I'd look, flat on my back on the grass as they started the race. I guess the humor of that image made me lose my nervousness. I was able to recover, get up and jog to the starting line.

—Tom Courtney, of the U.S., reflecting on his emotional state before winning the 800-meters final in the 1956 Melbourne Olympics

The feeling I get at the starting line is that it's over—all the hard work and training are over. The race is the fun part.

—Julie Moss, retired professional triathlete (courtesy of Ken Mierke of Evolution Running)

A Porsche that has run out of gas is no faster than a school bus that has run out of gas.

—Ken Mierke

Never take the lead unless you really want it, and if you take it, do something with it. Once in the lead, you have only two options, either you are going to pick up the pace, or you are going to slow it down. Once in control, a fast pace usually insures the fastest runner will win, a slow pace perhaps the fastest runner will still win but occasionally the race will go to the best kicker.

—Tom Courtney

It was a new kind of agony for me. It had never run myself into such a state. My head was exploding, my stomach ripping, and even the tips of my fingertips ached. The only thing I could think was, 'If I live, I will never run again!'"

—Tom Courtney

It's a shame for track and field. When I was the world record-holder, I ran against everyone. But now, people are scared of their reputations.

—John Walker, of New Zealand, won the 1,500-meters at the 1976 Montreal Olympics, and was first person to break 3:50 for the mile, setting a world record of 3min 49.4; he was also the first runner to break a four-minute mile 100 times (129)

The new Kenyans. There are always new Kenyans.

—Noureddine Morceli, of Algeria, and winner of the 1,500 meters at the 1988 Olympics, when asked if he feared any other runners

I can't understand how a guy can run so poorly between Olympics, and run so well at the Games. You have to give it to the guy. He must have some ability, but I think there's more to it than reindeer milk.

—Rod Dixon, on Lasse Viren

Let me tell you, Lasse Viren doesn't have to blood dope. Maybe the people he beats will have to do something, but not Lasse Viren. I've known him since he was 17, and he's simply the greatest distance runner in the world. But you see, Lasse Viren has four Olympic gold medals around his neck. The other runners only have excuses. That includes both Americans and New Zealanders, who have accused him of having some secret weapon. His secret is talent and hard training.

—Arthur Lydiard

The body does not want you to do this. As you run, it tells you to stop but the mind must be strong. You always go too far for your body. You must handle the pain with strategy. It is not age; it is not diet. It is the will to succeed.

—Jacqueline Gareau, 1980 Boston Marathon champion

The wreath or death!

—Athletes' oath during ancient Olympics

When you're at the starting line, the last thing you think about is money. When you're at the finish line, it's the first thing you think about.

—Rod Dixon

A short sprint is run on nerves. It's tailor-made for neurotics.

—Sam Mussabini, British track coach featured in *Chariots of Fire*

And now in one hour's time I will be out there again. I will raise my eyes and look down that corridor—four feet wide, with ten lonely seconds to justify my whole existence. But will I?

—Harold Abrahams, British sprinter in *Chariots of Fire*

Why couldn't Pheidippides have died here?

—Frank Shorter's comment to Kenny Moore at the 16-mile mark in an early career marathon for Shorter

The only tactics I admire are do-or-die.

—Herb Elliott

I wanted that record today. This means everything to me, to run on the track where Steve Prefontaine, one of my childhood heroes, ran.

—Alan Webb, on breaking the U.S. high school mile record (3:53.43), has the current national record of 3:46.91

WINNING

Winning

At what cost and personal sacrifice is victory ultimately measured? How would you answer that question? In 1967, Dr. Gabe Mirkin, who went on to write the best-selling The SportsMedicine Book, *asked competitive runners at a Washington, D.C., road race, "If I could give you a pill that would make you an Olympic champion — and also kill you in a year — would you take it?" Over half of the 100 runners who filled out the questionnaire responded that they would take the pill. (Morpheus from the movie,* The Matrix, *would have had his hands full with this crowd.)*

In our Vince-Lombardized sports culture, winning has tightened its hold on our collective athletic psyche. Running is not immune from this belief system. Competition is especially fierce at not only the super-elite level but among age-group race warriors. But for the majority of runners, victory is defined in a much less external, and more personal way: a finisher's T-shirt, shiny medal, new PR, weight loss, or improved health. Still, it's instructive and interesting to hear from the very best runners on what it means to win.

I've written history, pretty much. I just blew my mind and blew the world's mind.

—Usain Bolt, after setting world records in all three sprinting events at the Beijing Olympics (100 meters, 200 meters, 4×100 meters relay team)

I wasn't bragging. When I saw I wasn't covered, I was just happy.

—Bolt, on explaining why he started celebrating his victory 15 meters *before* reaching the 100-meters finish

We have to see it in the glory of their moment and give it to them. We have to allow the personality of youth to express itself.

—Jamaican government minister Edmund Bartlett, on defending Bolt's action in the wake of criticism by Olympic officials

If you want to win a race you have to go a little berserk.

—Bill Rodgers

I was scared of someone coming up on me. I didn't want it taken away. I could taste the third win.

—Bill Rodgers, on winning the 1978 Boston Marathon

After Boston, I was never quite the same. I had a few good races, but everything became difficult. Workouts that I used to fly through became an ordeal. And eventually, of course, I got so sick that I wondered if I'd ever get well.

—Alberto Salazar, on his 1982 marathon victory in 2:08:52

I'm never going to run this again.

—Grete Waitz, after winning her first of nine New York City Marathons

When I came to New York in 1978, I was a full-time school teacher and track runner, and determined to retire from competitive running. But winning the New York City Marathon kept me running for another decade.

—Grete Waitz

"You, sir, are the greatest athlete in the world."
"Thanks, King."

—Exchange between Gustav V of Sweden and Jim Thorpe at the 1912 Olympics

The man who can drive himself further once the effort gets painful is the man who will win.

—Roger Bannister

The reason sport is attractive to many of the general public is that it's filled with reversals. What you think may happen doesn't happen. A champion is beaten, an unknown becomes a champion.

—Roger Bannister

I am too tired, even to be happy.

—Gelindo Bordin, of Italy, immediately after winning the 1988 Olympic Marathon in Seoul

I was unable to walk for a whole week after that, so much did the race take out of me. But it was the most pleasant exhaustion I have ever known.

—Emil Zatopek, on his Olympic Marathon win in Helsinki in 1952

The battles that count aren't the ones for gold medals. The struggles within yourself—the invisible, inevitable battles inside all of us—that's where it's at.

—Jesse Owens

With victory in hand, running at maximum effort becomes very difficult.

—Frank Shorter

The medal is not for yourself. It couldn't be done without the support and help of my people, runners, and coaches.

—Alberto Juantorena, of Cuba, won both the 400 meters and 800 meters at the 1976 Olympics, and later served as the Vice Minister of Sports for Cuba

It's much more difficult staying on top than getting there.

—Robert de Castella

There is no formula for how many wins, records, or medals a runner must earn to qualify as "a legend." Rather, the sobriquet is reserved for those who carry a mystique that transcends the finish line, making them much more than champion athletes.

—Michael Sandrock

All my life people have been telling me, 'You're too small, Pre,' 'You're not fast enough, Pre,' 'Give up your foolish dream, Steve.' But they forget something: I have to win.

—Steve Prefontaine

I got caught in Seoul, lost my gold medal, and I'm here to tell people in this country it's wrong to cheat, not to take it, and it's bad for your health. I started taking steroids when I was nineteen years old because most of the world-class athletes were taking drugs.

—Ben Johnson, of Canada, whose 100-meters Olympic victory was nullified because of doping

I am very happy I got the gold medal; it had been my dream for years. To tell you the truth, I wasn't expecting to win. I thought I could reap a medal, but to win? Never. The world elite was all there, very strong girls, and I had never expected to defeat them and win the gold medal.

—Constantina Dita Tomescu, 38, of Romania, and the oldest Olympic women's marathon winner

Harold Abrahams: "If I can't win, I won't run! "
Sybil Gordon: "If you don't run, you can't win."

—from *Chariots of Fire*

I've known the fear of losing but now I am almost too frightened to win.

—Harold Abrahams, in *Chariots of Fire*

I am very satisfied for now. Please don't ask me about breaking 1:40!

—Wilson Kipketer, of Kenya, to reporters after setting a new world record in the 800 meters—a distance he dominated in competition for a decade

It is like a dream come true, I tell the journalists after the race. One of them later writes that this seems too hackneyed to describe such an emotional occasion. Well, what does he expect after a world record? Shakespeare?

—Brendan Foster, of England, after setting a 3,000 meters world record in 1974

I lost my first race at school and I was so jealous when the winner received a puppet that I said to myself, "I will carry on until I win a puppet."

—Svetlana Masterkova, of Russia, gold-medalist in the 800 and 1,500 meters at the 1996 Olympics

The victory took the stamp of eccentricity off me. I was a real athlete. My running had been looked upon as a diversion before.

—Frank Shorter, after winning the
1972 Olympic Marathon in Munich

New York is the one you have to win.

—Rod Dixon, winner of the 1983 New York City Marathon

The Games are littered with people who had one good day and were never heard of or seen again.

—Sebastian Coe, of England, winner of the
1,500 meters in the 1980 and 1984 Olympics

If I had to choose between a gold medal and a happy family life, I'd take the good family life every time.

—Ron Clarke

There's a lot of pressure to keep my record sparkling—no silvers or bronzes.

—Michael Johnson, winner of eight gold medals at
World Championships, and four Olympic gold medals
(200 meters, 400 meters, and 4 x 400 meters relay)

The only one who can beat me is me.

—Michael Johnson

I will always be the guy with the hat. The [golf cap] is more memorable than I am. It actually beats me into the Track and Field Hall of Fame by three years. Thinking back to Munich, I could take the high ground and say the 800 worked out just like I wanted, but in reality it was close to a disaster for me. I thought I could win the race, but I was so far behind from the gun that it shook my confidence. As it turned out, I was able to maintain the same pace while everyone else faded badly at the end.

—Dave Wottle, of U.S., and gold medalist in the 800 meters at the 1972 Summer Olympics

Now that I have run that time, I can say I have the ability to improve and go faster. I am very happy. It feels great to have the world record.

—David Lekuta Rudisha, of Kenya, on setting the fastest time ever in the 800 meters in 2010 (1:41:09)

Medals are nice, but they are only symbols.

—Emil Zatopek

I'm going to go out a winner if I have to find a high school race to win my last race.

—Johnny Gray, U.S. world-caliber 800-meters specialist who won a bronze medal at the 1992 Barcelona Olympics

First is first, and second is nowhere.

—Ian Stewart, of Scotland, winner of the 5,000 meters at the 1969 European Championships in 1969

Besides, a medal is only a thing, an object. The race, the achievement, is what's most important. I think the medal is still on the floor of my car—among the diapers.

—Joan Nesbit Mabe , after missing the World Indoor Championship 3,000 meters awards ceremony to return home to her two-year-old daughter

I remember winning a race at Salem (Massachusetts), and they gave me a pair of shoes – leather, business-type shoes for a professional to wear to a job. I took them and walked away, and an old geezer came up and said, 'You know you can't accept these shoes, don't you? You'll jeopardize your opportunity to run in the Pan American Games.' The shoes were worth more than $35, and that was the limit then. More than $35, and you were a professional.

—John J. "Young John" Kelley, Boston Marathon champion in 1957

I ran a race in Montreal once and won a refrigerator. It was the craziest race I'd ever run. Twenty-six miles in a ballpark, 118 times around the field!

—John A. "Old John" Kelley

When I knew I was going to win in 2004, I still felt awful. The last mile, I was just managing how much I was going to die.

—Alan Culpepper, winner of the 2004 U.S. Olympic Marathon Trials

Second place is not a defeat. It is a stimulation to get better. It makes you even more determined.

—Carlos Lopes, winner of the 1984 Olympic Marathon in Los Angeles, at age 37

I ran the race of my life, 2:08:53. Alberto happened to run two seconds faster. All I know for certain is that I left everything I had out on that course. I didn't give an inch. Neither did Alberto. The way I look at it, there were two winners that day.

—Dick Beardsley, on the 1982 Boston Marathon

That's not Frank! That's not Frank. It's an imposter! Get that guy off the track! How can this happen in the Olympic Games? It's bush league; get rid of that guy; there is Frank Shorter; that's Frank; come on, Frank, you won it. I wonder what Frank Shorter is thinking.

—ABC Sports commentator Erich Segal at the 1972 Munich Olympics, when a young German pretending to be Shorter ran onto the track

What I notice about the Olympics now, part of the human interest aspect of it, implied or overt, is the kind of loss of future income that comes from a failure or for not winning. It's so apparent now. . . . [A]t Munich, that was not how the Olympics were viewed. The goal was to be the best in the world on that particular day.

—Frank Shorter

I look at victory as milestones on a very long highway.

—Joan Benoit Samuelson

I made the school team, and when I won in a match against another school it was the greatest moment of my life—even greater than the European titles. In those school races, I always ran my legs off. There were girls watching and I wanted to impress them. I was foaming and vomiting, but I won.

—Juha Väätäinen, of Finland, winner of the 5,000-meters and 10,000-meters at the 1971 European Championships

It wasn't enough for me to win the race. I wanted to bury the other guys.

—Alberto Salazar

Roger, you only become really friendly with your opponents after you've beaten them!

—Don Macmillan, Australian miler, to Roger Bannister

Coming off the last turn, my thoughts changed from 'One more try, one more try, one more try...' to 'I can win! I can win! I can win!'

—Billy Mills, winner of the 10,000 meters at the 1964 Tokyo Olympics; his time of 28:24.4 was almost 50 seconds faster than his own PR and set a new Olympic record

Once my daughter asked if she could take my Olympic gold medal to school for "Show and Tell." I said that she could. Then I was curious about what she might say, so I showed up in her classroom that day and sat in the back. My daughter got up before the class and held up my medal and said: 'This is just like the medal Peggy Fleming won for ice skating.'"

—Billy Mills

All it takes is one totally obsessed guy and you'll be second every time.

—Scott Molina, one of the most dominant triathletes of the 1980s (courtesy of Ken Mierke of Evolution Running)

After I left the podium in Atlanta, I felt so fulfilled in my career that I lost my desire to compete at that level again.

—Carl Lewis, after winning the long jump at the 1996 Atlanta Olympics, where he won his ninth gold medal dating back to 1984; he retired the following year

He rubs it in too much. A little humility is in order. That's what Carl [Lewis] lacks.

—Edwin Moses, two-time Olympic gold medalist in the 400-meters hurdles

Even as [Joan] Benoit won the first women's Olympic marathon in 1984, I knew she was a legend. I tried to see such rare creatures as exemplars of the humanly possible, templates for the generations.

—Kenny Moore

Success is not measured in how fast you can run. It's measured in you doing your best and making improvements—then you are a success. You don't have to win the Olympics to be a success.

—Joe Douglas, Santa Monica Track Club coach and founder

The last mile was a cross between savoring the moment and just being really grateful that I was almost done.

—Shalane Flanagan, after winning the 2012 U.S. Olympic Marathon Trials and beating the previous Trials record by about three minutes

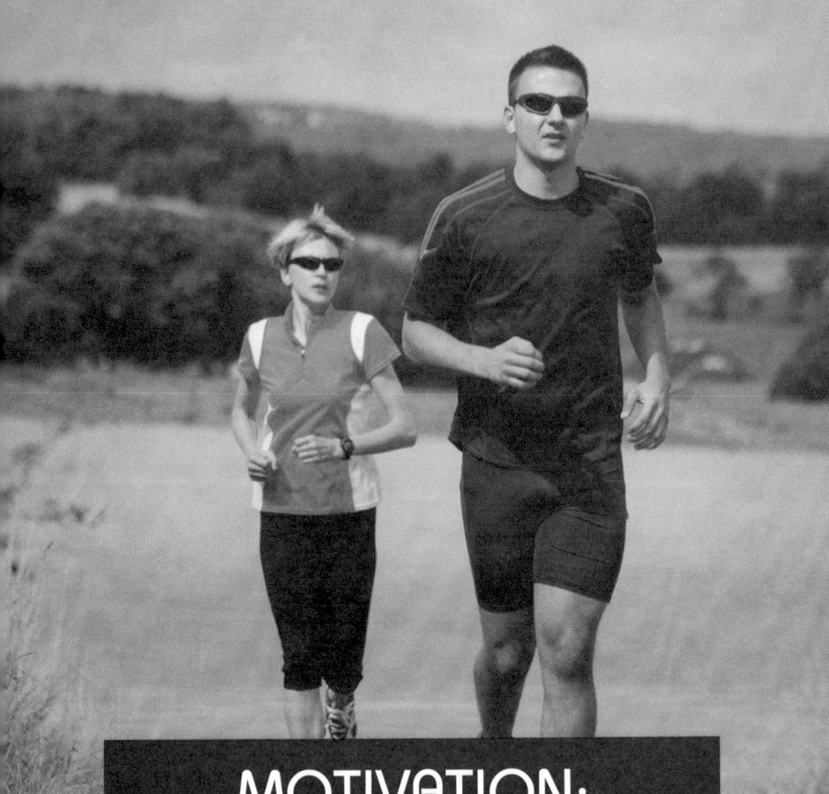

MOTIVATION: POSITIVE THINKING

Motivation is a sly fellow. A real slippery eel. Just when you think you have a firm grip on motivation, life's many distractions will rudely intrude and then to your personal dismay, you start wondering why regular workouts have suddenly become sporadic or regrettably a thing of the past. So it takes additional willpower and self-discipline to keep one's training on track, to ensure that one stays ahead of the procrastination game. That's why setting specific training or racing goals are critical for long-term success.

In a recent Runner's World *reader's poll, one of the questions asked, "What do you most want to improve?" Over 4,500 respondents answered as follows: 43 percent wanted to better their race times; 27 percent wished to increase their endurance; another 15 percent were looking at health benefits; 12 percent were focused on diet; and just 3 percent wanted to work on their attitude.*

Often times, you might feel burned out and in need of a break from running. By all means, take it. Refresh your mental batteries. But don't go slack. Stay active with say hiking, biking, or swimming. Researchers have found that after twelve weeks of no exercise, a highly trained athlete will have squandered a significant amount of fitness and conditioning. This equates to losing muscle mass, blood volume, and $V0_2$ *max of up to 20 percent. "Detraining" or deconditioning can be a downer. And should you have a running injury, try to find ways to remain physically active. Now let's see how some top runners have found ways to rev up their motivation. But first this, an amusing quote I once read in the* San Francisco Chronicle*: "Of course I'm not motivated. I'm paying you to motivate me"—client to personal trainer, overheard at a 24 Hour Fitness gym.*

The records fell easily at first. Dozens of seconds peeled away with every running of a course, and I could hardly wait for the next chance to improve.

—Joe Henderson

If you can train your mind for running, everything else will be easy.

—Amby Burfoot

Motivation is what gets you started. Habit is what keeps you going.

—Jim Ryun

My father told me it was not a job, that I wouldn't make a living at tennis . . . The toughest part was trying to explain to him that I could be the first one from Morocco to do it. But he didn't want me to play. We didn't talk for a year. That was when I knew I couldn't fail. I had to show him it was the right decision. It was a great motivation.

—Hicham El Guerrouj

Time marches on and here I am way up in my 80s. Jeepers. I want to run till I'm 100. I'll never stop. People ask me about my philosophy of life all the time. I just put one foot in the front of the other and keep going.

—John A. "Old John" Kelley, from *Young at Heart;* two-time winner of the Boston Marathon, which he finished 58 times

Average runners often use racing as one of the goals in their training. Maybe it is to help them continue through their training, maybe it motivates them to get out there on a consistent basis.

—Frank Shorter

The most important thing in the Olympic Games is not to win but to take part, just as the most important thing in life is not the triumph but the struggle.

—Baron de Coubertin, founder of the modern Olympics

If you need help getting motivated, turn to fellow runners. Often, they have been there, done that and can help move you along.

—Hal Higdon

You can't talk yourself into shape. Either you can do it or you can't.

—Frank Shorter

The five S's of sports training are: stamina, speed, strength, skill, and spirit; but the greatest of these is spirit.

—Ken Doherty

Running with others can help get you out when you might otherwise blow it off.

—Frank Shorter

Running in your dreams may also symbolize the energy levels, the strength, or the force that you have to get through life.

—Silvana Amar, *The Bedside Dream Dictionary*

To keep motivated, I started swearing at my husband for getting me into this mess in the first place.

—Grete Waitz on her first time running the New York City Marathon, in 1978

They say you can't run away from your troubles. I say that you can.

—John Bingham

When you've trained as best you can and you know your competition has done the same, nothing really matters but your mental strength and your belief.

—Florence Griffith Joyner

As I have aged, my running times and goals have changed, and so have my inspirations. I used to idolize the Olympic greats—the Paavo Nurmis, the Emil Zatopeks, the Abebe Bikilas, the Frank Shorters. Now I have a different hero—"Old John" Kelley, who has run the Boston Marathon sixty times.

—Amby Burfoot

It is the illusion that we can go no faster that holds us back.

—Kenny Moore

I've been asked if it's mental or physical ability that declines with age. I think it's mainly physical ability that changes, as opposed to any mental "burnout" that occurs from being at it for years.

—Bill Rodgers

Motivation is a skill. It can be learned and practiced.

—Amby Burfoot

The way I see it, you have to view running time not as extra or wasted time, but as important, productive contemplation time.

—Fred Lebow

Success is 90 percent physical and 10 percent mental. But never underestimate the power of that 10 percent.

—Tom Fleming

I don't know about psychology; I'm a runner.

—Steve Jones

Too many people have refused to begin running or have quickly dropped out of running programs because they "have no talent for it." Ridiculous. Talent has nothing to do with it. The only thing that matters is mental discipline.

—Amby Burfoot

Running isn't simply a discipline. It can become like a compulsion—it can become like a god. If you worship this god, you forget everything else. And when you lose this god, you've got nothing.

—Alberto Salazar

My upbringing gave me a strong will, a mental aggressiveness in what I wanted to achieve.

—Paul Tergat, of Kenya, held the world record in the marathon from 2003 to 2007, with a time of 2:04:55

Your toughness is made up of equal parts persistence and experience. You don't so much outrun your opponents as outlast and outsmart them, and the toughest opponent of all is the one inside your head.

—Joe Henderson

The greatest stimulator of my running career was fear.

—Herb Elliott

Is it raining? That doesn't matter. Am I tired? That doesn't matter, either. Then willpower will be no problem.

—Emil Zatopek

Running isn't simply a discipline. It can become like a compulsion—it can become like a god. If you worship this god, you forget everything else. And when you lose this god, you've got nothing.

—Alberto Salazar

I ran and ran every day, and I acquired a sense of determination, this sense of spirit that I would never, never, give up, no matter what else happened.

—Wilma Rudolph, winner of three gold medals in the 1960 Olympics (100 meters, 200 meters, and 4x100 meters relay)

I was pushed by myself because I have my own rule, and that is that every day I run faster, and try harder.

—William Kipketer

Most of the pressure I ever felt was self-imposed. I put a lot of pressure on myself. More than I should have, more than was healthy.

—Alberto Salazar

I raced supremely well. I felt I was as well fitted to do it as I had ever been, and as perhaps I might ever be. I went climbing three weeks before, because I was feeling fed up with running.

—Roger Bannister

When I am training and competing, I really concentrate, but during the rest of the day, I don't want to think about running.

—Ingrid Kristiansen, of Norway, four-time winner of the London Marathon and two-time winner of the Boston Marathon

Less inspired runners, including the vast majority of us, often find that they need some variety and excitement to get pumped up for their next workouts.

—Amby Burfoot

Once you're beat mentally, you might as well not even go to the starting line.

—Todd Williams, retired top American distance runner

Some Memorable Quotes from Several of the Shoe Giants

Happiness is pushing your limits and watching them back down.

—New Balance ad

There are clubs you can't belong to, neighborhoods you can't live in, schools you can't get into, but the roads are always open.

—Nike ad

Marathoning. The triumph of desire over reason.

—New Balance ad

A run begins the moment you forget you are running.

—Adidas ad

The only one who can tell you 'you can't ' is you. And you don't have to listen.

—Nike

Someone who is busier than you is running right now.

—Nike

But unless you are a runner, you won't understand.

—Nike

Training is the opposite of hoping.

—Nike

Some running should be different mentally, just the way it is different physically. On my easy runs, I may use the time to relax and let my mind wander, but I never do that in hard workouts or races.

—Grete Waitz

If I can get better, why not?

—Emil Zatopek

You can't climb up to the second floor without a ladder. When you set your aim too high and don't fulfill it, then your enthusiasm turns to bitterness. Try for a goal that's reasonable, and then gradually raise it.

—Emil Zatopek

Although this may seem like blasphemy to many racers, I suggest that your body, mind, and spirit will benefit from taking every fifth year of your running career as a retreat or recovery from racing. Take the year off from racing and just run for fun.

—Richard Benyo, editor of *Marathon & Beyond* and author of *Timeless Running Wisdom*

We all have dreams. But in order to make dreams into reality, it takes an awful lot of determination, dedication, self-discipline, and effort.

—Jesse Owens

I learned, one, you shouldn't ever quit. And I learned, two, you'll never be able to explain it to anybody.

—Jim Ryun

The difference between my world record and many world-class runners is mental fortitude. I ran believing in mind over matter.

—Derek Clayton

Accept the ups and downs you will experience. You are going to have days you feel like you're flying and days you struggle. This is normal for all runners.

—Grete Waitz and Gloria Averbach, *Run Your First Marathon*

You can be compulsive until your first big orthopedic injury. Once you have that, you begin to think more.

—Frank Shorter

Dream barriers look very high until someone climbs them. Then they are not barriers anymore.

—Lasse Viren

Great people and great athletes realize early in their lives their destiny, and accept it.

—Percy Cerutty

Wisdom Through the Ages

Study the past if you would define the future.

—Confucius

Fortune favors the brave.

—Virgil

Strength does not come from physical capacity. It comes from an indomitable will.

—Mahatma Gandhi

Nothing can withstand the power of the human will if it is willing to stake its very existence to the extent of its purpose.

—Benjamin Disraeli

You may fetter my leg, but Zeus himself cannot get the better of my free will.

—Epictetus, ancient Greek philosopher

No great thing is created suddenly.

—Epictetus

Difficulties are things that show a person what they are.

—Epictetus

First say to yourself what you would be; and then do what you have to do.

—Epictetus

They can conquer who believe they can. He has not learned the first lesson is life who does not every day surmount a fear.

—Ralph Waldo Emerson

The man who goes farthest is generally the one who is willing to do and dare. The sure-thing boat never gets far from shore.

—Dale Carnegie

Not being able to govern events, I govern myself, and apply myself to them, if they will not apply themselves to me.

—Michel de Montaigne, *Essays*, 1588

Discipline weighs ounces, regret weighs tons.

—Author Unknown

Man is never more human than when he plays.

—Friedrich von Schiller

The cyclone derives its powers from a calm center. So does a person.

—Norman Vincent Peale

If passion drives you, let reason hold the reins.

—Benjamin Franklin

Great souls have wills . . ...feeble ones have only wishes.

—Chinese Proverb

He who talks more is sooner exhausted.

—Lao Tsu

Do not wait to strike till the iron is hot; but make it hot by striking.

—W.B. Yeats

Never stand begging for that which you have the power to earn.

—Miguel de Cervantes

Be who you are and say what you feel, because those who mind don't matter and those who matter don't mind.

—Dr. Seuss

Man is not made for defeat. A man can be destroyed but not defeated.

—Ernest Hemingway

To improve is to change; to be perfect is to change often.

—Winston Churchill

Success consists of going from failure to failure without loss of enthusiasm.

—Winston Churchill

One must have a good memory to be able to keep the promises one makes.

—Frederick Nietzsche

One has attained to mastery when one neither goes wrong *nor hesitates* in the performance.

—Frederick Nietzsche

Be what you know you are.

—Pindar, ancient Greek poet

A graceful and honorable old age is the childhood of immortality.

—Pindar

Man needs difficulties; they are necessary for health.

—Carl Jung

You're not a man, you're a machine.

—George Bernard Shaw

The only way to define your limits is by going beyond them.

—Arthur Clarke

We can't all be heroes because someone has to sit on the curb and clap as they go by.

—Will Rogers

The secret of success is making your vocation your vacation.

—Mark Twain

THE PAIN GAME

I have never been good at playing the pain game. I'm not sure if this is due to some inherent defect in my character, or if the pain receptors in my brain are total wimps. The sprawling network of neurons and neural connections seem like a balky lot of French surrender monkeys, inclined to toss in the white flag early on.

So why are some runners better equipped at pain management than others? Even with lungs and legs besieged by a five-alarm fire of oxygen-debt, they are somehow able to push through the agony and discomfort. Total mystery, huh?

It's way too simplistic to chalk up athletic excellence as the logical outcome of the "no pain, no gain" conviction that is hard-wired into our jock being. But if you want to place high or win your age-group in the local 10K or half-marathon, you need to make that Faustian pact with the Pain Monster.

Almost all the world's top runners are exceptionally adept when it comes to masking their inner, red-lining agony. Perhaps they don't want their competitors to know how bad they are really suffering. So it's kind of a double whammy: you're in pain and you can't show it. The apt word to employ in this context is "stoic." It comes from the Greek word that means an indifference to pleasure or pain. An entire school of philosophy grew up around the suffer-in-silence concept.

Many centuries later, Freud became a student of the dynamic interplay between pain and pleasure. His view of the pleasure-pain principle suggested that we choose to obtain immediate gratification of our needs, which bring forth positive feelings of pleasure. The opposite is also true, and here the pain principle says that we consciously seek to avoid pain.

Could this be why we are addicted to running, with pleasure and pain jostling for supremacy like cage-bound mixed martial artist fighters? It's often the anticipation or delayed gratification of pleasure that allows us to soldier through the minefields of pain during a race. It's of some consolation knowing that once you get to the other side of the finish line, the battle is over. It makes the earlier suffering bearable.

But there is one kind of pain that should never be taken lightly. Runners do die in marathons, usually from heat exhaustion, electrolyte imbalance, water over-intoxication, or cardiac arrest. The message here is to always use common sense. If your body is telling you to quit, then quit.

Run like hell and get the agony over with.

—Clarence DeMar, winner of seven Boston Marathons, beginning in 1910

Pain is inevitable, Suffering is optional

—Haruki Murakami

I was always a great bundle of energy. As a child, instead of walking, I would run. And so running, which is a pain to a lot of people, was always a pleasure to me because it was so easy.

—Roger Bannister

You get very tired, and there was a certain amount of pain and you slow up. Your legs are so tired that you are in fact slowing. If you don't keep running, keep your blood circulating, the muscles stop pumping the blood back and you get dizzy.

—Roger Bannister

Learn to run when feeling the pain: then push harder.

—William Sigei, of Kenya, and former world-record holder in the 10,000 meters (26:52:23)

I was now running for the tape, the mental agony of knowing I had hit my limit, of not knowing what was happening behind me. I was not to know they were fading, too.

—Sebastian Coe

[H]is talent was his control of his fatigue and his pain. His threshold was different than most of us, whether it was inborn or he developed it himself.

—Walt McClure, on Steve Prefontaine

Thrust against pain. Pain is the purifier.

—Percy Cerutty

'No pain, no gain' does not mean that pain systematically equals gain. It's easy to go hard. It's hard to go smart.

—Erwan Le Corre

The social myth and competitive peer pressure associated with "no pain, no gain"—an attitude that "more is better" regarding more speed, more distance, more weights, and so forth—poses both fitness and health problems. Because when you're fully engaged in this approach, you override your brain's common sense—its instincts and intuition—to slow down during training. Making a conscious effort to go against what the brain wants to do can contribute to overtraining, often with an accompanying injury.

—Dr. Phil Maffetone

He loved the ache that shrouded his torso and he even waited for the moment, a few minutes into the run, when a dull voltage would climb his body to his brain like a vine, reviving him.

—Richard Christian Matheson, "Third Wind"

No pain, no Spain.

—Popular saying among athletes prior to 1992 Barcelona Olympics

The fear of running a long race can come from the fact that you know it's going to be physically painful. And unless you are a masochist, nobody likes pain. And if you dwell on this, it can make you nervous.

—Ron Hill on the marathon

It's at the borders of pain and suffering that the men are separated from the boys

—Emil Zatopek

I never felt as bad as I did over those last two miles. It was like running with a hangover.

—Geoff Smith, on finishing second (by nine seconds) to Rod Dixon in the 1983 New York City Marathon

Top results are achieved only through pain. But eventually you like this pain.

—Juha Vaatianen

The way I get through pain during a race is by telling myself everybody else is enduring worse.

—Dr. Steve Gangemi, aka "Sock Doc," and 17-time Ironman finisher

The only thing of which I am certain is that I have a greater capacity for punishment this season.

—John Landy, of Australia, and second runner to break four minutes in the mile

Racing is pain, and that's why you do it, to challenge yourself and the limits of your physical and mental barriers. You don't experience that in an armchair watching television.

—Mark Allen, six-time Hawaii Ironman winner

You hear it over and over again—a television announcer saying, "Watch that guy, he looks so relaxed." It's a rare athlete who wins who doesn't look relaxed.

—Mark Allen

I felt my throat start to close up, and I didn't think I was getting enough oxygen. I was scared, and I thought about quitting. But you don't want to quit when you've trained so hard and long for one race.

—Deena Kastor, on describing the effects of being stung by a bee in the back of the throat 100 meters after the start of the World Cross-Country Championships in Portugal. Despite blacking out and falling during the 8k race, she finished in twelfth place.

People think I'm crazy to put myself through such torture, though I would argue otherwise. Somewhere along the line we seem to have confused comfort with happiness. Dostoyevsky had it right: 'Suffering is the sole origin of consciousness.' Never are my senses more engaged than when the pain sets in. There is a magic in misery. Just ask any runner.

—Dean Karnazes, ultramarathoner whose feats of endurance are chronicled in several of his popular memoirs.

In football, you might get your bell rung, but you go in with the expectation that you might get hurt, and you hope to win and come out unscathed. As a distance runner, you know you're going to get your bell rung. Distance runners are experts at pain, discomfort, and fear. You're not coming away feeling good. It's a matter of how much pain you can deal with on those days. It's not a strategy. It's just a callusing of the mind and body to deal with discomfort. Any serious runner bounces back. That's the nature of their game. Taking pain.

—Chris Lear, author of *Running with the Buffaloes: A Season Inside with Mark Wetmore, Adam Goucher, and the University of Colorado Men's Cross-Country Team*

The Hawaii Ironman never lets you off easy. Especially the marathon. The calf pain in my left leg radiated up to my knee, worsening as I approached the halfway point along the hot lava highway. I shuffled forward like a demented, peg-legged Ahab, marking progress by the aid stations every mile. I was close to the airport. I wanted to just call it quits and take a cab back into Kona. (I had a $20 bill in my fanny pack.) I tried shifting my weight onto my right leg. That only worked to a limited degree, since it hurt every time my left shoe hit the road. I then attempted some visualization by mentally isolating Pain as the letter P within a Zen-like thought triangle. Mind over matter. The searing calf pain migrated inside the border of the triangle's three lines. Pain was now geometrically locked away in its prison cell. I was its jailer. It would not escape or defeat me.

—Bill Katovsky, 1982 Hawaii Ironman finisher

Checking in with Pain Experts

Behind every beautiful thing, there's some kind of pain.

—Bob Dylan

I assess the power of a will by how much resistance, pain, torture it endures and knows how to turn to its advantage.

—Frederich Nietzsche

There is no coming to consciousness without pain.

—Carl Jung

Pain is temporary. It may last a minute, or an hour, or a day, or a year, but eventually it will subside and something else will take its place. If I quit, however, it lasts forever.

—Lance Armstrong

After great pain, a formal feeling comes. The Nerves sit ceremonious, like tombs.

—Emily Dickinson

Satisfaction consists in freedom from pain, which is the positive element of life.

—Arthur Schopenhauer

Endure and persist; this pain will turn to good by and by.

—Ovid

In the country of pain we are each alone.

—May Sarton

If it doesn't work out there will never be any doubt that the pleasure was worth all the pain.

—Jimmy Buffet

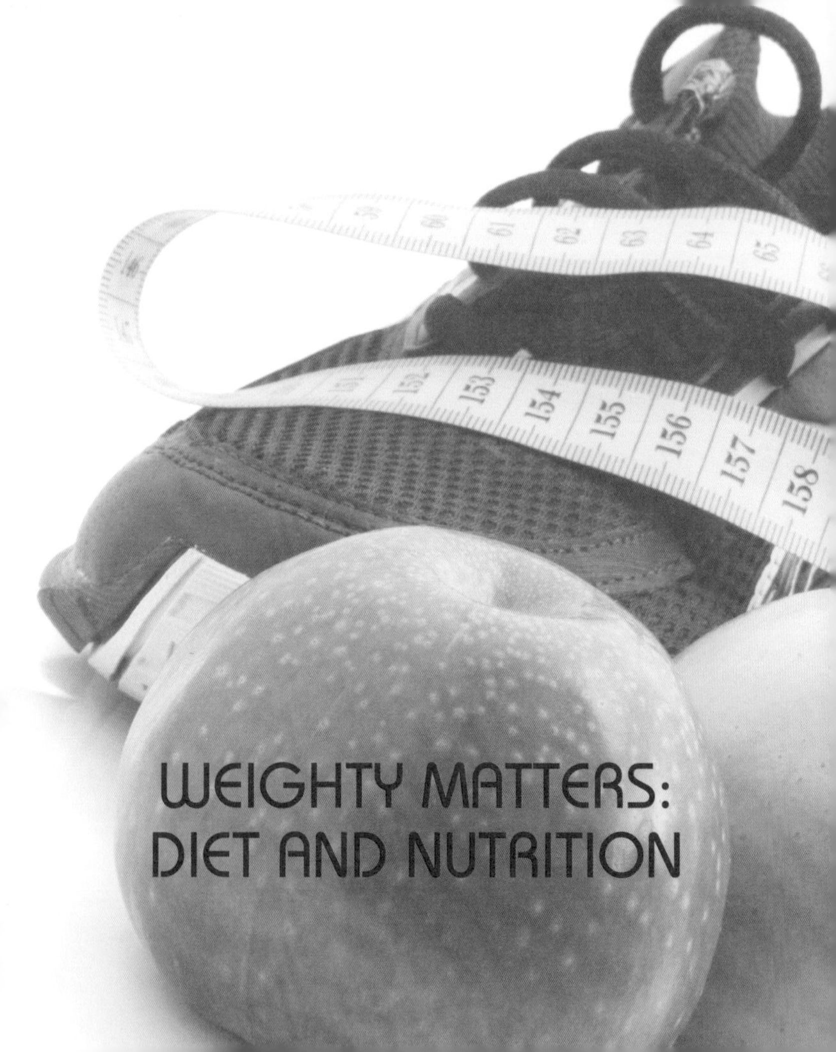

WEIGHTY MATTERS: DIET AND NUTRITION

It's really no secret that junk food plays a large role in running, more than is commonly acknowledged or discussed. Unhealthy food and beverages are often disguised in the form of high-fructose energy drinks, sugar-fortified energy bars, and all-you-can-eat pre-race pasta banquets where runners feel that they should eat like kings and queens. Yet for many runners, there is a tendency to overlook critical aspects of a poor diet, or wonder why they are still overweight with all the mileage they log—and while maintaining an obsession with comparing ounces when buying new running shoes.

Tom Osler, a top ultrarunner in the 1960s who later became a math professor and author of The Serious Runner, *conducted a comprehensive study of runners and found that for every extra pound one carries, that person will be 2.5 seconds per mile slower. If one is carting 10 extra pounds of belly fat, our marathon runner will be going 25 seconds slower per mile; it will take him an extra 11 minutes to finish the marathon! Plus, his heart, lungs, and muscles will have been working harder since he has more body mass.*

The ideal weight and optimal fat-to-lean ratio varies considerably for men and women as well as by age. The average adult body fat is 15 to 18 percent for men and 22 to 25 percent for women. The minimum percent of body fat considered safe for good health is 5 percent for males and 12 percent for females. Runners tend to be at the low end due to their increased lean weight, or muscle mass. Elite marathoners can have as low as 3 percent body fat. When Frank Shorter (five feet, ten inches) won the Olympic gold medal in the marathon in 1972, he weighed just 135 pounds with an alarmingly low body fat of 2.2 percent.

Just remember this: you don't need to be whippet-thin like the East Africans runners, but you can easily lose those extra stubborn pounds by following a sensible, healthy diet. Go heavy on fresh fruit, vegetables and lean protein, while staying clear of bad, high-glycemic carbs such as soft drinks, fruit juice, processed foods, bagels, corn, pasta, and potatoes. Watch your times drop with your weight. You will also feel better and have more energy. Diet isn't a zero-sum game of calories-in versus calories-out. It's where those calories come from that makes the real difference.

In the late 1960s and early '70s, almost every Sunday morning we'd go out for a hard 20-miler, then gulp down a huge quantity of orange juice or devour a whole watermelon. The term "electrolyte replacement drink" was unknown to us, and none of us carried a water bottle

—Ed Ayers

Coffee doesn't do it for me; it's running that gets me going.

—Joan Benoit Samuelson

All I want to do is drink beer and train like an animal.

—Rod Dixon

Prior to the 1991 New York City Marathon, I was walking down the street on the way to paint the blue line that runs along the course. I passed a pizza shop, and had a rare urge to indulge. It felt great. When it comes to food, I want to take advantage of every desire I have.

—Fred Lebow

What struck me most about Bill was that he would stop at every corner bakery and buy the gooiest pastries he could find, the kind with green frosting on them. He could eat anything.

—Pablo Vigil, one of the top mountain runners of the 70s, on Bill Rodgers

[As a *Sports Illustrated* writer] I cared more about evocative detail, about the image of an opal-pale [Bill] Rodgers, caught at 4:00 A.M. in the refrigerator's light after a 30-mile day, eating mayonnaise with a tablespoon from the jar, asking with perfect quizzicality, "Do I run so much to eat like this, or do I eat like this to run so much?"

—Kenny Moore

Let your running lead you to your diet.

—Bill Rodgers

Avoid any diet that discourages the use of hot fudge.

—Don Kardong

It wasn't that I was a glutton for punishment; it's just that my gluttony needed punishing.

—Bill Katovsky, prior to start of a 24-hour adventure race

A lot of times I'll tend toward a red meat type of thing, like a hamburger, because you can get a lot of calories really quickly. You know, put some mayonnaise on there. But you need that. You need some protein, you need some carbs, you need some fat. But also, for me, the sweet tooth comes into play. So there'll be a 7-Eleven fat boy run that night for after-dinner Kit Kats.

—Alan Webb, U.S. record-holder in the mile

His level of cooking is just beyond college dorm life. [Alan's] good with ramen noodles. You would think, he's some world-class athlete, he eats like brown rice and grilled chicken But nah, he'll eat like the greasiest Chinese food, and he'll eat like ice cream and cookies. He loves McDonald's. He ate a cheese steak with me a couple hours ago. He eats whatever he wants.

—Joe Zak, in a 2008 *Washington Post* interview with then-roommate of Alan Webb

As far as diet goes, Alan knows what works best. He went the ultra healthy disciplined route in previous years and it did not work. He does a great job getting a base of "healthy" stuff - fruits, good protein, dairy, etc.. but when you work out for 6 hours in a day, the most important thing is just getting the calories so you can come back strong the next day. Obviously its going to be hard to get in thousands of calories if you are only eating steamed broccoli and rice.

—Online comment by Webb's girlfriend and soon-to-be wife Julie Rudd in response to *Post* article

The walk finished, you will be more than ready for breakfast. This should, nevertheless, be a fairly light meal. Two or three medium-boiled eggs, a little fish, perhaps, some dry toast, and, say, two cups of coffee in preference to tea. It is as well to take some oatmeal porridge now and then in order to supply the necessary building material for one's bones, which is to be found in oatmeal in greater quantity than in any other food with which I am acquainted.

—Alf Shrubb, author and winner of 20 British distance titles between 1900 and 1904

I am firmly of the impression that the athlete who indulges in an occasional glass of [beer] will, other things being equal, derive greater benefits thereby than the man who preserves and adheres to a rigid teetotalism.

—Alf Shrubb

If you run 100 miles a week, you can eat anything you want - Why? Because: (a) you'll burn all the calories you consume; (b) you deserve it; and (c) you'll be injured soon and back on a restricted diet anyway.

—Don Kardong

The young man who meant to be a fast runner and tireless walker was enjoined to go through a course of physic taking, between an ounce and a half and two ounces of Glauber salts [laxatives] every four days until three doses had been administered.

—Walter Thom, top British "pedestrianism " (walker/runner) of the early 1800s

I eat whatever the guy who beat me in the last race ate.

—Alex Ratelle, U.S. masters running great who clocked 18 flat in the 5K at the age of 64

Eat food. Not too much. Mostly plants.

—Michael Pollan, *In Defense of Food*

How we eat, and even how we feel about eating, may in the end be just as important as what we eat. So we've learned to choose our foods by the numbers (calories, carbs, fats, R.D.A.s, price, what- ever), relying more heavily on our reading and computational skills than upon our senses. Indeed, we've lost all confidence in our senses of taste and smell.

—Michael Pollan, *The Omnivore's Dilemma*

Our over-reliance on grain-based nutrition is especially problematic.

—Loren Cordain, PhD, author of *The Paleo Diet*

The night before the race, we treated ourselves to a nice restaurant complete with a four-course meal of shrimp cocktail, baked potato, red wine, and ice cream.

—Grete Waitz, on the night before her first New York City Marathon win in 1978

One of the most popular and health-damaging diet plans is the low-fat diet.

—Dr. Phil Maffetone

Eggs are not just incredible, but what I would call the perfect food all wrapped up in one single cell. Yes, that's right, an egg is an individual cell. In this single cell, an egg contains the most complete and highest protein rating of any food, containing all essential amino acids.

—Dr Phil Maffetone

My favorite diet was a glass of beer with some bread and cheese.

—Walter George, late nineteenth century British running star

There are some runners who can train in Kenya, but I cannot. When I am in Kenya, the people invite me to drink tea with them, or to share food with them. And in my country, it is considered a great insult to refuse such an invitation So you see, I always gain weight when I visit Kenya, and it's difficult to stay in top condition. But in the U.S., I can concentrate on my training – and people must call me before they can come visit.

—Ibrahim Hussein, of Kenya, and three-time Boston Marathon champion

I consciously try to eat a lot of fresh, local fruits and vegetables, often purchased from the local farmer's market (April-November), but I definitely tend to eat a whole lot of straight-up carbs/sugar in the forms of pasta, breads, muffins, scones, cookies, Nutella on tortillas, chai, etc. I probably eat too much sugar. I don't eat any fast food, except for Illegal Pete's (local Chipotle-style burritos) here in Boulder, if that qualifies. In terms of eating enough to handle the mileage, I don't have a secret diet, however, I think I probably do have a fairly unique (i.e. slow) metabolism, because I don't feel like I eat a ridiculous amount. Or, maybe the quantity I eat is all I've ever known and it actually is a ridiculous amount. Or, maybe other people just eat too much relative to the amount of activity they have in their lives thereby making my diet not feel so out of place. I don't know.

—Anton Krupicka, U.S. top ultrarunner and two-time winner of the Leadville 100, from his blog

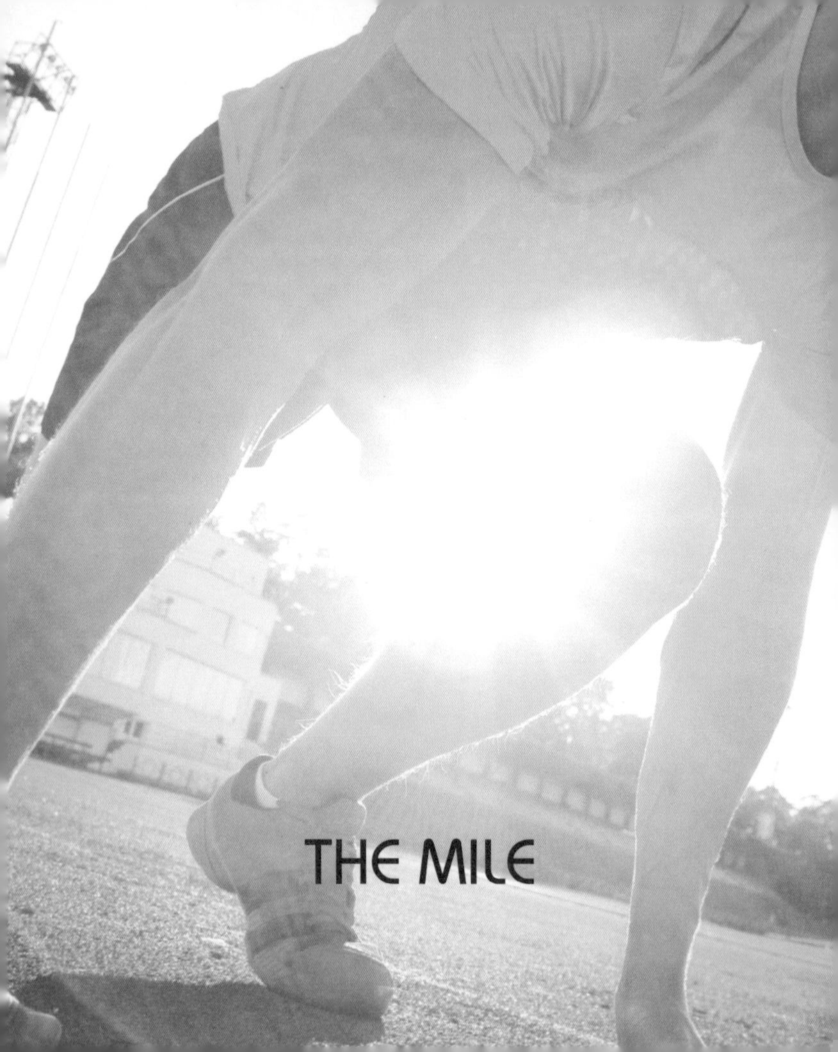

THE MILE

The Mile

The mile holds a strong emotional and physical attachment with almost all runners. The distance acts as our training and racing baseline, whether we log miles on the track, treadmill, or road. The current number of American runners who have broken four minutes in the mile is around 350; worldwide, that number jumps to 1,200. That figure could be much higher since the mile is not run as much as the 1,500 meters (also called the "metric mile") in international competition. (In the 1,500 meters, running 3:42.22 is equivalent to going 3:59.99 in the standard mile.)

So how did the mile come into being in the first place? The word is derived from the Latin or Roman word for mille, or 1,000, because a mile was the distance a Roman legion could typically march in 1,000 paces (or 2,000 steps, with a pace being the distance between successive falls of the same foot). And just how fast could Roman soldiers march? They typically had to cover 25 miles in five hours carrying a 70-pound backpack. His average pace would have been around eleven-and-a-half minutes-per-mile.

Since miles of varying lengths were used throughout Western Europe, in 1592, the British Parliament finally settled the question by defining the statute mile to be 8 furlongs, 80 chains, 320 rods, 1,760 yards or 5,280 feet.

That was the distance that Roger Bannister covered in 1954 on the Oxford, England, track when he clocked the very first sub-four minute mile. At the time, it seemed like an impossibly heroic feat, the human equivalent of a jet smashing through the sound barrier. But the world record for the mile was 4:01.4, which was set by the Swedish runner Gunder Haag in 1945. All Bannister really had to do was whittle away 1.5 seconds over four laps, or just under 4/10ths of a second every circuit.

Bannister ran the mile in 3 minutes and 59.4 seconds. His two pacesetters had positioned him well for a 59-second last lap. By his own estimation, Bannister said afterwards that he had run 20,000 miles in eight years of ceaseless preparation for the day of reckoning.

Seven weeks later, the Australian John Landy broke Bannister's record by going 3:58. The times have dropped ever since. Hicham El Guerrouj, of Morocco, holds the world record in 3:43.13. Ironically, Bannister, arguably the most famous miler, is also the man who held the world record for the shortest period of time.

By the way, I may be trying for the four-minute mile at Oxford soon.

—Roger Bannister in a letter to his sister Joyce

The mile has all the elements of drama.

—Roger Bannister

I found longer races boring. I found the mile just perfect.

—Roger Bannister

You cannot run a fast mile race if there is a strong wind, because it makes your running uneven.

—Roger Bannister

The Athletic Association competed against the University. So there was an event. You cannot break world records unless it is an established event, and you have three timekeepers, and the whole thing is organized.

—Roger Bannister

The art of taking more out of yourself than you've got.

—Roger Bannister on running the mile

If I faltered, there would be no arms to hold me and the world would be a cold and forbidding place.

—Roger Bannister

I knew you would do it one day, Roger.

—Roger Bannister's mother after he broke the four-minute mile

It is in fact only a time.

—Roger Bannister

Roger Bannister studied the four-minute mile the way Jonas Salk studied polio - with a view to eradicating.

—Jim Murray, *Los Angeles Times* sports columnist

I am not exceptionally disappointed. There still is the challenge to see who will be the first American to break the 4-minute mile.

—Wes Santee, one of the top U.S. milers in the early 1950s and former world record-holder in the indoor mile; his fastest time ever was 4:00.5

He was a pretty good guitar player. He used to play with a band until I told him he would have to choose between guitar and track. He couldn't do both and be a four-minute miler.

—Fred Dwyer, Marty Liqouri's high school coach

To run a world record, you have to have the absolute arrogance to think you can run a mile faster than anyone who's ever lived; and then you have to have the absolute humility to actually do it.

—Herb Elliott

A miler is the aristocrat of running. A miler is the closest thing to a thoroughbred horse that exists on two legs.

—John L. Parker, Jr., *Once a Runner*

First, I figured out the time I thought the mile should be run in. Second, I started testing my theories and particularly my own constitution and capabilities; the result of this study soon convinced me that the then existing records at the distance were by no means good.

—Walter George

Blink and you miss a sprint. The 10,000 meters is lap after lap of waiting. Theatrically, the mile is just the right length - beginning, middle, end: a story unfolding.

—Sebastian Coe

By breaking the world record every few days, those two Limeys are making a mockery of the mile race, which has traditionally been the core and kernel of any track meet.

—Red Smith, *New York Times* sports columnist, on Sebastian Coe and Steve Ovett

Frankly, I think the four-minute mile is beyond my capabilities. Two seconds may not sound much, but to me it's like trying to break through a brick wall.

—John Landy after running a 4:02 mile

The mile has a classic symmetry. It's a play in four acts.

—John Landy

[A]lmost every part of the mile is important—you can never let down, never stop thinking, and you can be beaten at almost any point.

—John Landy

[It gave me] equal pleasure as running 4:02 for the mile.

—John Landy on finding a stenciled hairstreak butterfly (he was a collector)

It was done. Finished. Next thing.

—John Landy, after setting the mile record

Landy had tried so hard, and I am very glad that he has now succeeded. It shows that times can always be broken.

—Roger Bannister, after Landy beat his mile record

Whether we athletes liked it or not, the 4-minute mile had become rather like an Everest: a challenge to the human spirit, it was a barrier that seemed to defy all attempts to break it, an irksome reminder that men's striving might be in vain.

—Roger Bannister

I think it is bloody silly to put flowers on the grave of the 4-minute mile, now isn't it? It turns out it wasn't so much like Everest as it was like the Matterhorn; somebody had to climb it first, but I hear now they've even got a cow up it.

—Harry Wilson, top British coach and one of the founder members in the early 1960s of the British Milers Club

There was nothing unusual about my victory. The entire story was back in eighth place. There is simply no way to imagine how good Jim Ryun is or how far he will go after he becomes an adult. What he did was more significant than Roger Bannister's first mile under 4 minutes.

—Dyrol Burleson, after winning the Compton Invitational Mile in 1964; Ryun, only 17, ran 3.59,0

The Mile

It was a fast time, especially for a drug-free mile. It's a very good time. So I was a little bit surprised but I knew what it took to do: it took a lot of hard work and I don't think there were too many people who worked as hard as me. It took someone with the talent — there have been people along the way who had talent but they didn't work hard. They trained like 800 (meters) runners and tried to run a mile and it didn't work. So it took someone (Alan Webb) with the talent, but someone who also wasn't afraid to work hard, and that is what Alan did.

—Steve Scott, in 2010 interview, on setting the American outdoor mile record (3:47.69), which stood for 26 years.

The race itself – my recollection is not so good, but the one thing I do remember is you can't see the finish line from the start line, but you come over a little hill and then you can see the finish, and it looked so close. I remember starting to kick because it looked like "oh, it's just a quarter-mile away," but in reality, it was probably over 800 meters away. I just totally ran out of gas because it looked like the finish line, instead of getting closer, kept getting farther and farther away with every step I took. From a tactical point of view, it was a difficult thing to adjust to. But from a social point of view, it was great because it was at the end of a season, it brought all the great milers together at one place, and it was a very social event. The Road Runners treated us like kings. We went out afterward to Studio 54.

—Steve Scott, in a 2010 *Runner's World* interview, on finishing seventh in the Fifth Avenue Mile in New York in 1981

The 800 meters record, the records in the 1000, the 1500, the 5000, the relays: no one remembers them. The mile, they remember. Only the mile.

—John Walker, of New Zealand, was the first person to run the mile in under 3:50 (1975)

That magical four-minute mile barrier has set a universal standard. To run under that time is a phenomenal achievement. For the average runner, to see how close that person can come to the "almighty" gives them an indication of where they really stand.

—Eamonn Coghlan

In certain ways, the feeling of running a mile in 3:49 is exactly the same as when I ran my first marathon in 2:25 in New York in 1991. And that sheer exhilaration that you experience is the same for a world-class runner as it is for a jogger.

—Eamonn Coghlan

Running a fast mile feels almost like you're flying like a bird, in complete control of everything that's going on, physically and mentally. You feel absolutely fantastic, like a runaway express train that could effortlessly go on and on forever.

—Eamonn Coghlan

I think everyone should try running a mile. People can relate to the mile.

—Eamonn Coghlan

In the moment of victory I did not realize that the inner force, which had been driving me to my ultimate goal, died when I became the world's fastest miler.

—George Derek Ibbotson, of England, who set a new world record (3:57.2) in 1957

Some Other Mile Records in Case You Want to Try

Somersaulting: 19 minutes, 11 seconds
Pogostick Jumping: 12 minutes, 16 seconds
Milk Bottle Balancing on Head: 7 minutes, 47 seconds
Hula Hooping: 11 minutes, 29 seconds
Tiddlywinks: 23 minutes, 22 seconds

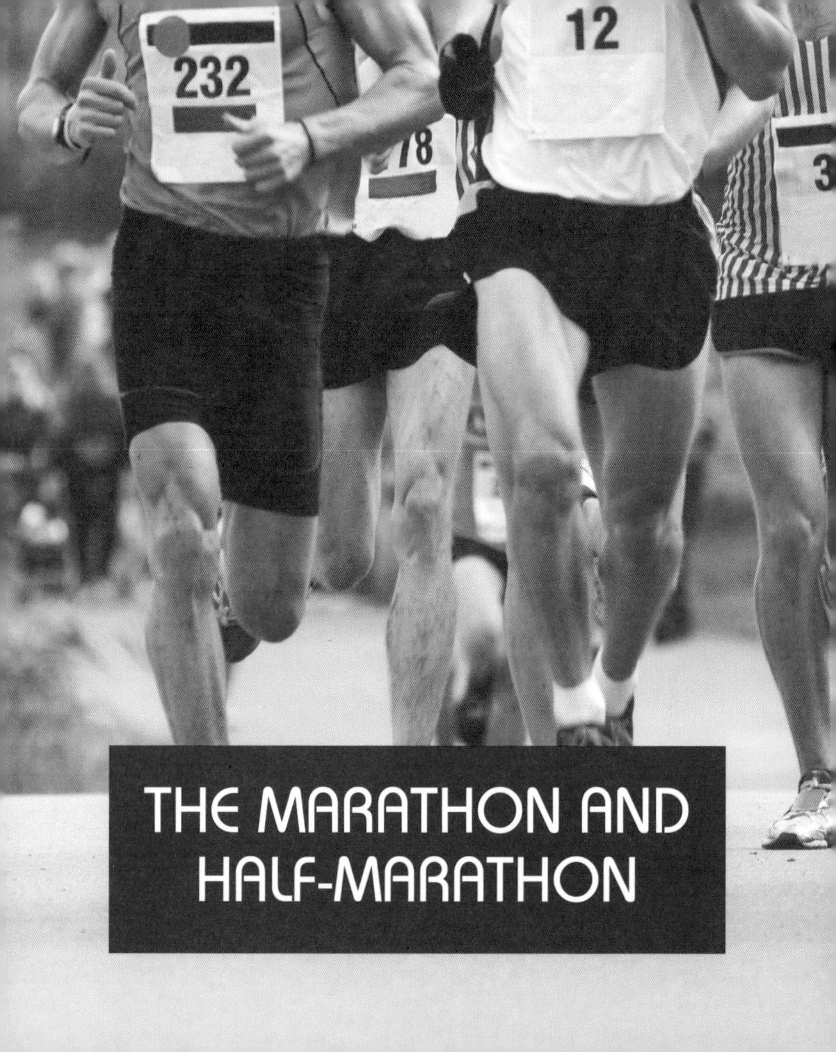

THE MARATHON AND HALF-MARATHON

Marathon mania is sweeping across America. Over 500,000 runners finished a marathon in 2010, according to a published report by Running USA. The half-marathon number is even more staggering: 1.4 million finishers. Since 2003, the half-marathon has been the fastest growing road race distance in this country, with women making up 59 percent of the field. In the full marathon, men comprise 59 percent of the field.

Running USA's Half-Marathon Report offered the following reasons for the increase in half-marathon runners: "The popularity of the distance has been fueled mainly by charity and non-charity training programs, destination-type events/series, runners moving up or down from the marathon and women's participation."

Because marathoners and half-marathoners are the ultimate number-crunchers, always thinking in terms of mile splits, minutes run per diem, PRs, training data logged into their favorite fitness apps, let's look at some other noteworthy statistics of 26.2 and 13.1.

- *In 1897, the first Boston Marathon (just under 25 miles) debuted one year after the Athens Games with just 15 starters. Ten runners finished. By 1902, the field swelled to 42 runners, with over 100,000 spectators lining the course.*

- *It wasn't until 1964 that more than 300 runners entered the Boston Marathon.*
- *In 1976, 25,000 runners finished a marathon in the U.S.*
- *The average age of a male marathon finisher today is 40; for women it's 36.*
- *The average finishing time of a male marathoner today is 4:27; for women it's 4:54.*
- *The top seven marathons in the U.S. based on the total number of 2010 finishers: New York City (44,704); Chicago (36,159), Boston (22,540), Los Angeles (22,403); Marine Corps (21,974); Honolulu (20,169); Disney World (16,874).*
- *In 2010, there were 664 official marathon finishes in the U.S. under 2:30, and more than 9,000 finishes under 3:00.*
- *The number of masters (40 years old and higher) who finished a marathon in 1980 in the U.S. was 10 percent; by 2010, the number increased to 46 percent.*
- *The number of juniors (under 20 years old) who finished a marathon in 1980 in the U.S. was 5 percent; by 2010,*

the number decreased to 2 percent.

- *Of the largest timed road race events in the United States, 42 percent of them are half-marathons.*
- *Since 1995, the number of female finishers in the half-marathon has increased by a factor of six (135,000 women in 1995 to 820,000 in 2010).*
- *Seven of the top 15 "women-only" events in the nation are half-marathons.*
- *Average age of a half-marathon finisher: men (39); women (36).*
- *Average time of a half-marathon finisher: men (2:00); women (2:19).*

I had as many doubts as anyone else. Standing on the starting line, we're all cowards.

—Alberto Salazar, winner of Boston and three New York City Marathons

Anything worth doing is going to be difficult.

—Fauja Singh, 100 years old, after finishing the 2011 Toronto Marathon in 8:25

The marathon can humble you.

—Bill Rodgers, ranked top marathoner in the world by *Track & Field News* in 1975, 1977 and 1979

I was unable to walk for a whole week after that, so much did the race take out of me. But it was the most pleasant exhaustion I have ever known.

—Emil Zatopek, on his marathon win (and third gold) at the 1952 Helsinki Olympics

If you want to run a mile, then run a mile. If you want to experience another life, run a marathon.

—Emil Zatopek

Know why people run marathons? Because running is rooted in our collective imagination, and our imagination is rooted in running. Language, art, science; space shuttles, Starry Night, intravascular surgery; they all had their roots in our ability to run. Running was the superpower that made us human.

—Christopher McDougall

I think the idea of a two-hour marathon is thoroughly ridiculous. Absolutely ridiculous.

—Derek Clayton

When a marathon was over, it was like a huge weight had lifted off my shoulders. I think that the best moment of a marathon was just afterward, soaking in the tub, with no more people around, no more expectations.

—Alberto Salazar

Since I'd read *Walden* in high school, I had been haunted by Thoreau's charge that when I came to die, I might discover that I had not lived. If I ran a marathon, I thought, I will have lived. I also thought I might die.

—Benjamin Cheever, author of *Strides*

He let the pack take him to 19 miles at perfect pace and he then found himself in the right place at the right time to move into the history books with an eyeballs-out, lung-busting, gut-wrenching six-mile surge to the finish.

—Charles Spedding, winner of the London Marathon, on Steve Jones's world record at the 1984 Chicago Marathon

I just run as hard as I can for 20 miles, and then race.

—Steve Jones, when asked about his racing strategy, after he had won the 1984 Chicago Marathon

I remember watching Frank Shorter in the [1972 Munich Olympic] marathon. But I wasn't thinking that I'd end up in the Olympics. It was so far away from that, and something I couldn't conceive of.

—Bill Rodgers

The marathon is a charismatic event. It has everything. It has drama. It has competition. It has camaraderie. It has heroism. Every jogger can't dream of being an Olympic champion, but he can dream of finishing a marathon.

—Fred Lebow, New York City Marathon co-founder and race director

When you first run up First Avenue in New York, if you don't get goose bumps, there's something wrong with you.

—Frank Shorter, on the New York City Marathon

I think I bit off more than I could chew, I thought the marathon would be easier. For the level of condition that I have now, that was without a doubt the hardest physical thing I have ever done.

—Lance Armstrong, after finishing the New York City Marathon for the first time in 2006, in 2:59

I would sooner be prime minister of the moon than run another marathon. I've been really lucky. I didn't have any toenails fall off or anything disgusting like that. I still have all three nipples.

—Ryan Reynolds, actor

As an actor, you spend your whole life pretending. Completing a marathon was the first time in my adult life I had done something that had a huge physical attachment to it. It required everything, not just my imagination."

—Anthony Edwards, actor

I actually had people running up next to me offering me shots. All of this crazy stuff. And no, I didn't take any of it.

—Will Ferrell, actor, on running the Boston Marathon

Never in my life have I ever experienced anything as crazy as this.

—Sean "P. Diddy" Combs, on finishing the 2009 New York City Marathon in 4:14:54

Twenty-six miles isn't a publicity stunt.

—Sean "P. Diddy" Combs

I'll never do that again!

—Grete Waitz, after winning the first of nine consecutive New York City Marathons

Everyone wins the marathon. We all have the same feeling at the start—nervous, anxious, excited. It is a broader, richer, and even with twenty-seven thousand people—more intimate experience than I found when racing in track. New York is the marathon that all the biggest stars want to win, but has also been the stage for an array of human stories more vast than any other sporting event.

—Grete Waitz

Knowing that you can run 20 miles is a big breakthrough mentally, when it comes to tackling the marathon distance.

—Joan Benoit Samuelson

When I run a marathon, I put myself at the center of my life, the center of my universe. For these hours, I move past ideas of food and shelter and sexual fulfillment and other basic drives.

—George Sheehan, M.D.

The marathon is charismatic. It has everything. It has drama. It has competition. It has camaraderie. It has heroism.

—Fred Lebow

All men may not be brothers, but that's the way it feels after a marathon. . . . you feel—you can't help but feel—that you all understand each other.

—Benjamin Cheever, *Strides*

Every serious marathoner should do Boston, to experience the close to a million spectators, the three generations of families out cheering, the little kids handing you water or orange slices. The whole city really appreciates the runners.

—Neil Weygandt, finisher of 41 straight Boston marathons as of 2011, with a PR of 2:36:51 in 1983

If people were possessed by reason, running marathons would not work. But we are not creatures of reason. We are creatures of passion.

—Noel Carroll, top Irish middle-distance runner of the mid-1960s

The marathon is like a bullfight . . . there are two ways to win. There's the easy way if all you care about is winning. You hang back and risk nothing. Then kick back and try to nip the leaders at the end. Or you can push, challenge the others, make it an exciting race, risking everything.

—Alberto Salazar

The marathon is the focal point of all that has gone before and all that will come afterward.

—George Sheehan, M.D.

It is important to keep the marathon in perspective. Running does not have to be the controlling element in your life, but if you become a marathon runner it probably will be, for a while.

—Marc Bloom, *The Runner's Bible*

The difference between the mile and the marathon is the difference between burning your fingers with a match and being slowly roasted over hot coals.

—Hal Higdon, "On the Run from Dogs and People"

Marathons are extraordinarily difficult, but if you've got the training under your belt, and if you can run smart, the races take care of themselves.

—Deena Kastor, first American woman to run a marathon under 2:20

I have been asked everywhere I go: Why do people run the marathon? Sure, there is a sense of status we gain among our peers. But I think the real reasons are more personal. I think it is because we need to test our physical, emotional, or creative abilities.

—Fred Lebow

It was a fantastic finish at the stadium. Everyone was on their feet clapping and we had a piper. It was a wonderful reception. I'm still on a bit of a high and I will probably still be on one tomorrow when I realize I don't have to get the suit on. Now I'm having a dram of whisky to celebrate.

—Lloyd Scott, after setting a new world record in 2003 for the slowest marathon time by finishing the Edinburgh Marathon in six days, four hours, 30 minutes and 56 seconds – while wearing a 130-pound, deep-sea diving suit

It is horrible, yet fascinating, this struggle between a set purpose and an utterly exhausted frame.

—Sir Arthur Conan Doyle, commenting on Italy's Dorando Pietri's collapse in the last 100 meters of the 1908 Olympic Marathon; because race officials helped him cross the finish line, he was stripped of the gold medal

It was impossible to leave him there, for it looked as if he might die in the very presence of the Queen.

—Official Olympic report on why officials helped Pietri across the line

Virgin charity runners who have never run a step are trained to run a marathon within six months. Often, when they line up at the starting line, they've never run another race on the way to attempting 26.2 miles and they are still 30 to 40 pounds overweight. The results are preordained: they run a marathon, they acknowledge that it was the most incredibly difficult physical thing they've ever done or are most likely to do, and they never run again. The athlete within never sees the light of day, and the romance of the marathon distance is undermined because it wasn't raced; it was survived. (This is not to say that all charity program coaches are inept. But if all of them were adept, there wouldn't be dozens – sometimes hundreds of charity runners out on a marathon race course long after the course closes.) These runners are cheated out of becoming *runners*.

—Richard Benyo, author of *Timeless Running Wisdom*

If you feel bad at 10 miles, you're in trouble. If you feel bad at 20 miles, you're normal. If you don't feel bad at 26 miles, you're abnormal.

—Rob de Castella, winner of 1983 World Marathon Championship

When I took my artificial right leg for a 26.2-mile run in 1976, I had no idea how it would change my life. I entered the New York City Marathon that year because I was a runner and that is what runners do. No other amputee had attempted to run a marathon before. The norms of society, and of sport, dictated that it was an impossible event, but I was soon to let it be known that it was, indeed, possible.

—Dick Traum, founder of the Achilles Track Club for disabled athletes

It was so thick with spectators you couldn't even see how the hills went up. It was just this mass of humanity, people hanging out of trees or whatever.

—Dick Beardsley, on the Boston Marathon crowds

The marathon is my only girlfriend. I give her everything I have.

—Toshihiko Seko, two-time winner of Boston Marathon and dominant long-distance runner in the 1980s

I was motivated to win [the Boston Marathon] not only for myself, but for the Portuguese people of Boston. They were with me all the way and made winning this race the nicest moment of my life.

—Rosa Mota, three-time winner of Boston Marathon and Olympic gold-medalist in Seoul (1988)

Running a marathon is 90 percent mental toughness. The rest is in your head.

—Anonymous

He didn't have the marathon bug. He didn't have the focus he developed later.

—Amby Burfoot, on his college roommate Bill Rodgers

Abebe planted the idea that the marathon could be raced in a different way. Up until then, people would save themselves, waiting to see who would drop. He helped change the tactics.

—Frank Shorter on Abebe Bikila

There is the truth about the marathon and very few of you have written the truth. Even if I explain to you, you'll never understand it, you're outside of it.

—Douglas Wakiihuri, speaking to journalists

The Boston Marathon has had more to do with liberating and promoting women's marathoning than any other race in the world.

—Joe Henderson

The marathon's about being in contention over the last 10K. That's when it's about what you have in your core. You have run all the strength, all the superficial fitness out of yourself, and it really comes down to what's left inside you. To be able to draw deep and pull something out of yourself is one of the most tremendous things about the marathon.

—Rob de Castella

Lisa: You got all your equipment, Dad?
Homer: Let's see. Sweatbands check, anti-chafing nipple tape check, check, and check.

—From *The Simpsons*, as Homer preps for the Springfield Marathon

You have to forget your last marathon before you try another. Your mind can't know what's coming.

—Frank Shorter

A half marathon is a good way to have a bit of fun and race against those girls and learn a bit more about them.

—Paula Radcliffe

I think the job toughened me up, climbing and walking and stooping all day. When I began my run at night, I was tired; but after a mile or so, the tiredness went away.

— Johnny Kelley, two-time Boston Marathon winner, on his job at Boston Edison Electric Company

Frank and Bill were both absolutely essential to the running boom, in completely different ways. Frank's biggest imprint was winning the Olympics. Frank was the Olympian in every sense, more regal, king of the land. Bill clearly was the boy next door.

—Amby Burfoot, on Frank Shorter and Bill Rodgers

There hasn't been a Boston Marathon since the two favorites ran together all the way from Hopkinton, doing everything possible to beat each other, neither one giving an inch. I think it was the greatest American distance race.

—Alberto Salazar, on the 1982 Boston Marathon "Duel in the Sun" with Dick Beardsley

Anyone can run 20 miles. It's the next six that count.

—Barry Magee, of New Zealand, bronze medalist in the marathon at the 1960 Rome Olympics

A lot of people have checked the marathon off their 'life list.' But they don't want running out of their lives.

—Ryan Lamppa, a spokesman for Running USA, a nonprofit organization that tracks trends in running, on the rise of half-marathons

We believe the half-marathon is the new hot distance. With the right course, the New York City Half could be as big or bigger than the marathon.

—Mary Wittenberg, the president of the New York Road Runners, which organizes the New York City Marathon and Half-Marathon

In 1971, the New York City Marathon was no bigger than a grade-school field day. It was the race's second year, and a shivering cult of 245 runners gathered in Central Park to run laps around the walking paths.

—Edward McClelland, author and journalist

The starting line of the New York City Marathon is kind of like a giant time bomb behind you about to go off. It is the most spectacular start in sport.

—Bill Rodgers, as a television commentator, in 1987

The half-marathon gives you almost all of the satisfaction and achievement of the marathon and far less than half of the aches and pains and fatigue.

—Jeff Galloway

The marathon has been referred to as a person's horizontal Everest.

—Grete Waitz and Gloria Averbach, *Run Your First Marathon*

[The half-marathon] has a niche of serious respectability. It's viewed as a real challenge on its own, so runners are more likely to feel content tackling it instead of the full marathon.

—Amby Burfoot

13.1 Miles: It isn't half of anything.

—slogan for nationwide 13.1 Marathon series

For somebody who is 53 and used to be fat, I thought that was really good. I'd never run a half-marathon before, and given what my diet and exercise used to be like, I was amazed that I even finished.

—Drew Carey, actor and host of *The Price is Right,* on completing the Marine Corps Half-Marathon in 1:57

What do I have to run to beat Oprah's time?

—popular Google search phrase; Oprah Winfrey ran a 4:29:20 in the 1994 Marine Corps Marathon; it was her first and only marathon

I'm running a lot of half-marathons. I'm content just to do halves right now.

—Bill Rodgers, in 2009, following the USA Master's Half-Marathon where he finished fourth in his age group in 1:34:16

Do you think I'm old. I feel like I am 20.

—Haile Gebrselassie, 37, then world-record holder in the marathon at a press conference on the eve of the 2010 New York City Marathon; an inflamed knee caused him to drop out of the race

Selections from @RunningQuotes Twitter feed

- *Good thing it's not 26.3 miles, because THAT would be insane.*
- *Sweat is sexy.*
- *Ice Bath and Cookies Ahead!*
- *Forget www.Match.com, I'm looking for a man that can go long.*
- *I bet this sounded like a good idea when you signed up 6 months ago.*
- *Free Nipple Massages*
- *You are NOT almost there.*
- *It's not sweat, it's your fat cells crying!*
- *Toenails are overrated.*
- *Do you still think this is a good idea?" (sign at mile 20)*
- *Momma said there'd be days like this.*
- *Some day you won't be able to do this. Today is NOT that day.*

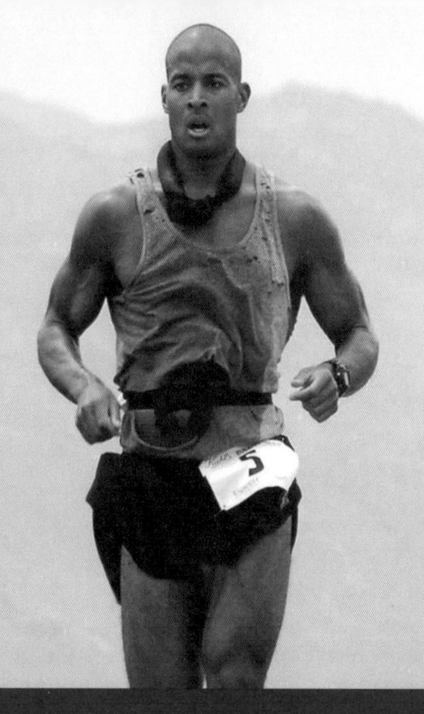

THE ULTRAMARATHON: GOING BEYOND 26.2

Just as the increased interest and participation in marathons has helped popularize its kid brother, the half-marathon, it's also fueled the recent growth of ultramarathons, or ultras. An ultra is any race over 26.2 miles, and can cover a broad range of distances and conditions, ranging from 50K affairs in urban parks to the six-day-long contest of 151 miles in the Sahara Desert known as the Marathon des Sables. It's estimated that over 70,000 runners worldwide annually compete in an ultra.

Another type of ultra is the 24-hour endurance run. The goal for competitors is to see how many miles they can run, walk, or hobble in the space of one day. The NorthCoast 24-hour event, now its third year and held in Cleveland near the shores of Lake Erie, is tailor-made for those who have physically and mentally come to terms with monotony. The race-course consists of a .90075-mile loop on a flat, ten-foot wide asphalt path. In 2011, Philip McCarthy, 43, of New York, won by legging out 153.37 miles; women's winner Connie Gardner, 47, of Medina, Ohio, covered 144.72 miles.

Scott Jurek, who many of us got to know by reading Born to Run, *owns the U.S. 24-hour record; he went 165 miles at a race in France in 2010. The world record is 178 miles, which belongs to Yiannis Kouros, of Greece. Another way to consider 178 miles: it's only several miles longer than the driving distance between Portland, Oregon and Seattle, Washington.*

But it's not as if one can show up on race day, sign an indemnification waiver, and charge off into the dawn with other fanny-pack-toting ultrarunners. One of the oldest and most demanding trail events in the U.S., The Western States Endurance Run (aka The Western States 100), starts high up in the Sierras at Squaw Valley, California, and ends in Auburn, California, a body-thumping total of 100 off-road miles. Runners climb a cumulative total of 18,090 feet and descend 22,970 feet. Those who finish under 30 hours receive a bronze belt buckle; under 24 hours will earn you a silver belt buckle to hold up your pants. The men's record is 15 hours and 7 minutes set by Geoff Roes in 2010; Ann Trason, who won the event a mind-boggling 14 times, established the women's record of 17 hours and 34 minutes in 1994.

Because The Western States 100 is held on U.S. Forest Service lands, the size of the field is limited to 369 runners. Which means that the demand far exceeds the supply of available race slots. A special lottery is held to select the majority of participants unless a runner has won a race in the Montrail Ultra Cup series. Each year, over 2,000 runners from around the world try their luck. That means the odds of being accepted are just north of 10 percent. Yet to be even eligible for the opportunity to have Lady Luck smile upon you, there are mandatory qualifying standards such as running 50 miles in under 11 hours.

A runner who's habitually attracted to ultras often appears to have the air of an endurance ascetic, like a secular Saint Francis of Assisi in shorts, singlet and trail-running shoes. Nothing better pleases these long-distance runners than finding himself or herself on a mountainous single-track path, hours from home, the next aid station, or finish line. Their fatigued bodies are on auto-pilot, with a quiet hush enveloping them in a moving cocoon of perpetual motion, the only sound being the soft, gentle crunch of their shoes nimbly finding their way on the narrow footpath.

Ultrarunners have plenty of time to think. Which makes their thoughts about running all the more interesting. Let's take a quick journey into the mind of the ultrarunner.

It hurts up to a point and then it doesn't get any worse.

—Ann Trason

People think ultra is some kind of spaghetti eating contest for people with no talent to do anything else.

—Ann Trason

The first fifty miles are run with the legs, the second fifty with the mind.

—Anonymous

The best long distance *runners* eat raw meat, run naked and sleep in the snow.

—Alaska Airlines advertisement, courtesy of ultrarunner Stan Jensen

So as we walked along the river toward Rucky Chucky, I said the words that most men say to a pretty woman as they walk along the river under a starry night on their first date: "If you were a real hardass, you'd stick your finger down your throat and clear your stomach and if you won't do it, I will."

—Stan Jensen, pacing Sarah Lowell at the 1997 Western States 100

"Why aren't you signed up for the 401K?"
"I'd never be able to run that far."

—from the Dilbert comic strip

The trail is well marked.

—Anonymous

You eat the elephant one bite at a time.

—Anonymous

From here, it's all downhill but the uphill.

—Anonymous

Speed is sex ... distance is love.

—David Blaike, Canadian ultrarunner

Perhaps the genius of ultrarunning is its supreme lack of utility. It makes no sense in a world of space ships and supercomputers to run vast distances on foot. There is no money in it and no fame, frequently not even the approval of peers. But as poets, apostles and philosophers have insisted from the dawn of time, there is more to life than logic and common sense. The ultrarunners know this instinctively. And they know something else that is lost on the sedentary. They understand, perhaps better than anyone, that the doors to the spirit will swing open with physical effort. In running such long and taxing distances they answer a call from the deepest realms of their being—a call that asks who they are.

—David Blaikie

At mile 80, it's not all that great, but you live through it and then fondly recall how good it was.

—Tim Twietmeyer, five-time winner of the Western States 100

There's no tangible reward in anything I do, certainly not in running Western States. It's just an interesting challenge.

—Tim Twietmeyer

Training to run 100 miles is like training to get hit by a truck.

—Luis Escobar, seven-time finisher of the Western States 100

A pure racing animal. The top ultrarunner in the country, maybe in the world, arguably of all time.

—Chris McDougall, on Scott Jurek in *Born to Run*; Jurek had seven consecutive wins at Western States 100 and was two-time winner of the Badwater Ultramarathon in Death Valley

Sometimes I wonder, am I being selfish? Running ultramarathons is a pretty selfish thing. It feels good to motivate people to run and take care of their bodies. But I wonder, am I serving a greater purpose?

—Scott Jurek

There are a lot of times it's just not fun. It's a lot of discomfort. There must be something I'm searching for.

—Scott Jurek, on why he runs

Running an ultramarathon is 90 percent mental; the other 10 percent—that's mental too,

—Scott Jurek

It's about finding one's path. It's about using experience in life to shape something completely different. That's the art of living.

—Scott Jurek

Beware of the chair!

—Anonymous

The race continued as I hammered up the trail, passing rocks and trees as if they were standing still.

—Red Fisher, on his Wasatch Front 100 run in 1986

Surprisingly, the "idea" of running a hundred miles didn't frighten me. Instead, it awakened in me a curiosity, a wonder in myself, my ability, my strength, both physical and mental, and a quiet want. I simply let it live inside me for a while, months, a year, two years, until I felt it coming out as stronger than just a murmur.

—Kris Whorton, elite female masters ultrarunner

If you start to feel good during an ultra, don't worry you will get over it.

—Gene Thibeault, ultrarunner

The thing I don't like about Western States is that you show up at the starting line in the best shape of your life and a day later you are in Auburn in the worst shape of your life.

—Andy Black, ultrarunner on Western States 100

You're not puking and nothing's broken so get going.

—Vivian McQueeney to her husband, Scott, in the middle of the climb to Whitney Portal during the Badwater Ultramarathon in Death Valley

You can be out there having your worst day, but at the same time the person next to you is having their best day. So there's really no room for crankiness in the sport. At least I try to minimalize it.

—Suzie Lister, on The Western States 100

When you are 99 miles into a 100-mile race, your brain is not the same brain you started with.

—Paul Huddle, multisport coach and former professional triathlete

We (ultrarunners) alternate between depression and stupidity.

—Don Kardong

In an ultra you should eat like a horse, drink like a fish, and run like a turtle.

—Anonymous

Run when you can, walk if you have to, crawl if you must; just never give up.

—Dean Karnazes, author of the bestselling *Ultramarathon Man: Confessions of an All-Night Runner;* and 11-time finisher (under 24 hours) of the Western States 100

How to run an ultramarathon? Puff out your chest, put one foot in front of the other, and don't stop till you cross the finish line.

—Dean Karnazes

I run because long after my footprints fade away, maybe I will have inspired a few to reject the easy path, hit the trails, put one foot in front of the other, and come to the same conclusion I did: I run because it always takes me where I want to go.

—Dean Karnazes

Unless you're not pushing yourself, you're not living to the fullest. You can't be afraid to fail, but unless you fail, you haven't pushed hard enough.

—Dean Karnazes

Some seek the comfort of their therapist's office, other head to the corner pub and dive into a pint, but I chose running as my therapy.

—Dean Kaernazes

Sometimes you've got to go through hell to get to heaven.

—Dean Karnazes

The Leadville 100 is like running the Boston Marathon twice with a sock in your mouth and then hiking to the top of Pikes Peak. Now that you have done that, turn around and do it all over again in the dark.

—Christopher McDougall

At first, the idea of running in circles for 24 hours sounds crazy. But I think it was much, much more fun than a typical loop or point-to-point race. You get to see people many times over those 24 hours, whereas in a different race, you may see them once.

—Comment on NorthCoast 24's Facebook Page

Relentless Forward Progress.

—Anonymous

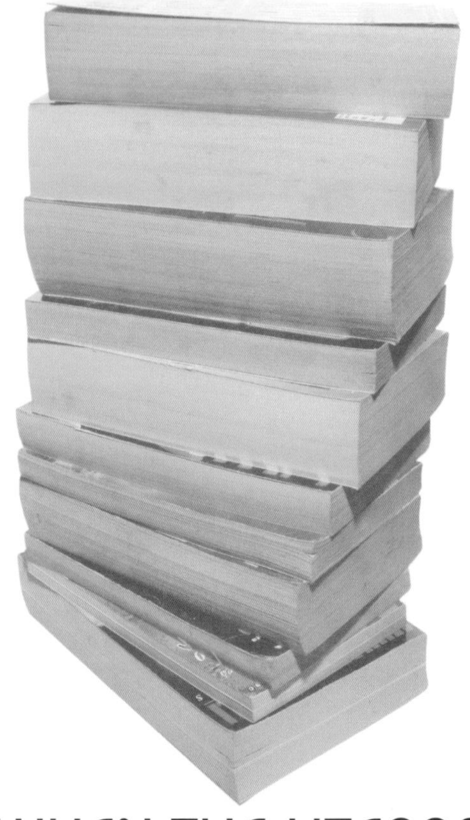

WHEN THE LITERARY CANON GOES OFF

Running has a stealth-like, beneath-the-radar relationship with literature. Unlike modern sports such as football, baseball, or golf that have produced countless novels and short stories, running lacks that marquee rapport with fiction writers and their readers. Most runners who came of age during the first running boom have heard about (and possibly read) both of these two running-based classics, The Loneliness of a Long Distance Runner *and* Once a Runner*; but one can probably assume that very few new runners have actually read either one.*

I read Loneliness shortly after I started running in 1980, and was less than impressed by the plot, main character, or even the author, Alan Sillitoe's writing style. The short story about a young, rebellious working-class British bloke who has a gift for speed left me with the same "so what?" attitude that I got after finishing A Separate Peace, *which is rammed down almost every student's gullet in eighth or ninth grade.*

Because of that lackluster experience, I never bothered giving John L Parker's novel a chance, despite the critical raves it received from serious runners. In fact, before the 1978 title was re-issued as a reprint in 2010, Once a Runner *was the top-selling used book on Bookfinder.com.*

Competitive runners emotionally bonded with Quenton Cassidy as a true-to-life symbol of what it took to become a top miler – the fire in the belly, monastic lifestyle, lung-scalding and leg-burning track workouts, take-no-prisoners approach to racing. It was all there for thoroughbred runners to say to themselves, "I can identify. That's me *on the page!"*

Literature's grand aim is exhuming deep, universal truths about human toil, sacrifice, fate, character, and choices made and their ultimate consequences. Running seems like the ideal medium to explore these hard-fought truths. Fortunately, if you look long enough or know where to begin searching, you will eventually realize that running has been hiding all along in plain sight within the boundaries of literature. Verses about running are found in the Bible. The ancient Greek poets celebrated athletes of the Olympic Games. Shakespeare occasionally got in on the act, as did modern masters like James Joyce and Ernest Hemingway.

This chapter opens up only a small window to this rich literary world. For further immersion in the subject, I heartily recommend Roger Robinson's excellent, insightful and highly readable Running and Literature, *which is also the source for over a dozen passages that appear in this section. Robinson is an English scholar and New Zealand-based elite runner with over 50 years of racing. Along with numerous masters victories in long-distance races all over the globe, he placed first in the masters division at the 1984 Boston Marathon in a time of 2:20:15. He's married to Kathrine Switzer, the real-life heroine for women runners.*

Perhaps, someday an author will write a modern novel based on the Greek mythological figure, Atalanta, the beautiful princess who was known for winning footraces against potential male suitors. If they lost (and they all did except for the cunning Hippomenes who tricked her with three golden apples), the defeated men were put to the sword.

Of prizes in the games thou art fain, O my soul, to tell, then, as for no bright star more quickening than the sun must thou search in the void firmament by day, so neither shall we find any games greater than the Olympic whereof to utter our voice: for hence cometh the glorious hymn and entereth into the minds of the skilled in song, so that they celebrate the son of Kronos, when to the rich and happy hearth of Hieron they are come [. . .]

—Pindar, ancient Greek lyric poet

Great runner, four times victor at the Games. But for a war you would have known no fame. Though exiled from the bubbling springs of home, Your swift pace made a new land's fields your own.

—Pindar

When the Literary Canon Goes Off

You quick Greek, Aglaus,
you earned the wild applause
you stirred and fuelled
that filled Poseidon's field
with roars.
Out of the groove you moved
as fire burns a field
and up the track you ran and spun
around the turn
and back and then
again and then again
without a pause
for breath, you ran
to rising noise
with springy poise,
the men behind
like panting boys.

—Bacchylides, ancient Greek poet

Now bid me run,
And I will strive with things impossible,
Yea, get the better of them.

—Shakespeare, *Julius Caesar*

Great Akhilleus, hard on Hektor's heels,
kept after him, the way a hound will harry
a deer's fawn he has startled from its bed
to chase through gorge and open glade, and when
the quarry goes to earth under a bush
he holds the scent and quarters till he finds it;
so with Hektor: he could not shake off
the great runner, Akhilleus.

—Homer, *The Iliad*

On a flat road runs the well-train'd runner;
He is lean and sinewy, with muscular legs;
He is thinly clothed—he leans forward as he runs,
With lightly closed fists, and arms partially rais'd.

—Walt Whitman, "The Runner"

Run naked, goaded sore by wasps and hornets,
A swarm that stung the more the wretches fled.

—Dante's *Inferno,* Canto 3

Thus, though we cannot make our sun
Stand still, yet we can make him run.

—Andrew Marvell, "To His Coy Mistress"

Swift of foot was Hiawatha;
He could shoot an arrow from him,
And run forward with such fleetness,
That the arrow fell behind him!
Strong of arm was Hiawatha;
He could shoot ten arrows upward,
Shoot them with such strength and swiftness,
That the tenth had left the bow-string
Ere the first to earth had fallen!
He had mittens, Minjekahwun,
Magic mittens made of deer-skin;
When upon his hands he wore them,
He could smite the rocks asunder,
He could grind them into powder.
He had moccasins enchanted,
Magic moccasins of deer-skin;
When he bound them round his ankles,
When upon his feet he tied them,
At each stride a mile he measured!

—Henry Wadsworth Longfellow, "The Song of Hiawatha"

The true competitive runner, simmering in his own existential juices, endured his melancholia the only way he knew how; gently, together with those few others who also endured it, yet very much alone.

—John L. Parker, Jr., *Once a Runner*

It is simply that we can all be good boys and wear our letter sweaters around and get our little degrees and find some nice girl to settle, you know, down with . . .Or we can blaze! Become legends in our own time, strike fear in the heart of mediocre talent everywhere! We can scald dogs, put records out of reach! Make the stands gasp as we blow into an unearthly kick from three hundred yards out! We can become God's own messengers delivering the dreaded scrolls! We can race black Satan himself till he wheezes fiery cinders down the back straightaway!

—from John L Parker's *Once a Runner*

Gazalla ed aquila
Il silenzio
dell'altopiano
Il boato all' stadio
("Gazelle and eagle/The silence/The plateau/The cheering in the stadium.")

—Aldo Rossi, an Italian poet, on Abebe Bikila

Now, here, you see, it takes all the running you can do, to keep in the same place. If you want to get somewhere else, you must run at least twice as fast as that.

—Alice, speaking in Lewis Carroll's *Through the Looking-Glass*

But he ran on—uphill, and downhill, the same pace alike –like the shadow of a cloud.

—Thomas Hardy, from his first novel *Desperate Remedies*

Do something that involves use of the body. How can you hope to run when you spend the whole day standing still? How can you hope to master your own body when your body is the slave of a machine?

—Brian Ganville, from the short story "The Olympian"

To An Athlete Dying Young, by A. E. Housman, from A Shropshire Lad (1896)

The time you won your town the race
We chaired you through the market-place;
Man and boy stood cheering by,
And home we brought you shoulder-high.

Today, the road all runners come,
Shoulder-high we bring you home,
And set you at your threshold down,
Townsman of a stiller town.

Smart lad, to slip betimes away
From fields where glory does not stay
And early though the laurel grows
It withers quicker than the rose.

Eyes the shady night has shut
Cannot see the record cut
And silence sounds no worse than cheers
After earth has stopped the ears:

Now you will not swell the rout
Of lads that wore their honour out,
Runners whom renown outran
And the name died before the man.

So set, before its echoes fade,
The fleet foot on the sill of shade,
And hold to the low lintel up
The still-defended challenge-cup.

And round that early-laurelled head
Will flock to gaze the strengthless dead,
And find unwithered on its curls
The garland briefer than a girl's.

Women have more stamina. I knew it before liberation.

—Nurse Phillips, from Max Apple's short story "Carbo-Loading"

They knew him only as another of those crazy runners who goes out every day to punish himself into a state of fitness. And to give the dogs and the motorists fits.

—Bruce Tuckman, from the short story "Long Road to Boston"

I can't go on, I'll go on.

—Samuel Beckett

Run when I can, walk when I cannot run, and creep when I cannot walk.

—John Bunyan, Pilgrim's Progress (1678)

We swing ungirded hips
And lighten'd are our eyes,
The rain is on our lips,
We do not run for prize.
We know not whom we trust
Nor whitherward we fare,
But we run because we must
Through the great wide air.

—Charles Hamilton Sorley, "The Song of the Ungirt Runners"

Out came the children running.
All the little boys and girls,
With rosy cheeks and flaxen curls,
And sparkling eyes and teeth like pearls,
Tripping and skipping, ran merrily after
The wonderful music with shouting and laughter.

—Robert Browning, "The Pied Piper of Hamelin"

Still as they run they look behind,
They hear a voice in every wind,
And snatch a fearful joy.

—Thomas Gray, "Ode on a Distant
Prospect of Eton College"

If you can force your heart and nerve and sinew
To serve your turn long after they are gone,
And so hold on when there is nothing in you
Except the Will which says to them: "Hold on!"

—Rudyard Kipling, "If "

The wind is old and still at play
While I must hurry upon my way,
For I am running to Paradise;
Yet never have I lit on a friend
To take my fancy like the wind
That nobody can buy or bind.

—William Butler Yeats, "Running to Paradise"

I had the road all to myself, and I fairly flew—leastways I had it all to myself except the solid dark, and the now-and-then glares, and the buzzing of the rain, and the thrashing of the wind, and the splitting of the thunder; and sure as you are born I did clip it along!

—Mark Twain, *The Adventures of Huckleberry Finn*

Men, wives, and children stare, cry out, and run,
As it were doomsday.

—Shakespeare, *Julius Caesar*

Why dost thou run so many mile about?

—Shakespeare, *Richard III*

Go, run, fly and avenge us.

—Pierre Corneille, *The Cid* (1636)

If you had but looked big and spit at him, he'd have run.

—William Shakespeare, *The Winter's Tale*

At Marathon arrayed, to the battle shock we ran
And our mettle we displayed, foot to foot, man to man
And our name and fame shall not die.

—Aristophanes, *The Acharnians*

Like wine through clay,
Joy in his blood bursting his heart,
He died—the bliss!

—Robert Browning, "Pheidippides"

I remember the way he'd pull on a rubber shirt over a couple of jerseys and a big sweat shirt over that, and get me to run with him in the forenoon in the hot sun... "Come on kid," he'd say, stepping up and down on his toes in front of the jock's dressing room, "let's get moving."

—Ernest Hemingway, from the short story "My Old Man"

But those who wait on the Lord Shall renew their strength;
They shall mount up with wings like eagles,
They shall run and not be weary
They shall walk and not faint.

—Isaiah 40:31

Know ye not that they which run in a race run all, but one receiveth the prize? So run, that ye may obtain. And every man that striveth for the mastery is temperate in all things. Now they do it to obtain a corruptible crown; but we an incorruptible. I therefore so run, not as uncertainly; so fight I, not as one that beateth the air: But I keep under my body, and bring it into subjection: lest that by any means, when I have preached to others, I myself should be a castaway.

—I Corinthians 9:24-27

Then would begin Stephen's run around the park. Mike Flynn would stand at the gate near the railway station, watch in hand, while Stephen ran around the track in the style Mike Flynn favored, his head lifted high, his knees well lifted and his hands held straight down by his sides.

—James Joyce, from
Portrait of the Artist as a Young Man

North of Laguna, two Zuni runners sped by them, going somewhere east on "Indian business . . . They coursed over the sand with the fleetness of young antelope, their bodies disappearing and reappearing among the sand dunes, like the shadows that eagles cast in their strong, unhurried flight."

—Willa Cather, from the novel
Death Comes for the Archbishop

House Master: So, uh, how do you come to be here?
Colin Smith: [*puzzled*] I got sent, didn't I?
House Master: [*chuckles*] Yes, I know you got sent, but why?
Colin Smith: I got caught. Didn't run fast enough!

—Alan Sillitoe, *The Loneliness of the Long Distance Runner*

If any of you want tips about running, never be in a hurry, and never let any of the other runners know you are in a hurry even if you are.

—Alan Sillitoe, *The Loneliness of the Long Distance Runner*

The two men ran, pursuer and pursued,
and he who fled was noble, he behind
a greater man by far. They ran full speed,
and not for bull's hide or a ritual beast,
or any prize that men compete for; no,
but for the life of Hektor, tamer of horses.

—Homer, *The Iliad*

I would give a thousand pound. I could run as fast as thou canst.

—Falstaff to Poins in Shakespeare's *Henry IV*

We may outrun. By violent swiftness that which we run at,
And lose by over-running.

—Shakespeare, *Henry VIII*

The Tortoise and the Hare, from Aesop's Fables (1911 translation by Edward Plunkett)

For a long time there was doubt with acrimony among the beasts as to whether the Hare or the Tortoise could run the swifter. Some said the Hare was the swifter of the two because he had such long ears, and others said the Tortoise was the swifter because anyone whose shell was so hard as that should be able to run hard too. And lo, the forces of estrangement and disorder perpetually postponed a decisive contest.

But when there was nearly war among the beasts, at last an arrangement was come to, and it was decided that the Hare and the Tortoise should run a race of five hundred yards so that all should see who was right.

"Ridiculous nonsense!" said the Hare, and it was all his backers could do to get him to run.

"The contest is most welcome to me," said the Tortoise,

"I shall not shirk it."

O, how his backers cheered.

Feeling ran high on the day of the race; the goose rushed at the fox and nearly pecked him. Both sides spoke loudly of the approaching victory up to the very moment of the race.

Then they were off, and suddenly there was a hush.

The Hare dashed off for about a hundred yards, then he looked round to see where his rival was.

"It is rather absurd," he said, "to race with a Tortoise." And he sat down and scratched himself. "Run hard! Run hard!" shouted some.

"Let him rest," shouted others.

And after a while his rival drew near to him.

"There comes that damned Tortoise," said the Hare, and he got up and ran as hard as could be so that he should not let the Tortoise beat him.

The Hare ran on for nearly three hundred yards, nearly in fact as far as the winning-post, when it suddenly struck him what a fool he looked running races with a Tortoise who was nowhere in sight, and he sat down again and scratched.

"Run hard. Run hard," said the crowd, and "Let him rest."

"Whatever is the use of it?" said the Hare, and this time he stopped for good. Some say he slept.

There was desperate excitement for an hour or two, and then the Tortoise won.

When the Literary Canon Goes Off

The town talk this day is of nothing but the great foot-race run this day on Banstead Downes, between Lee, the Duke of Richmond's footman, and Tyler, a famous runner. And Lee hath beaten him; though the King and Duke of York and all men almost did beat three or four to one upon the Tyler's head."

—Samuel Pepys's diary, July 30, 1663

The boy's face was ash-pale and his lips, wrenched back from his teeth, were white. He was cotton-mouthed, racking for breath, but he was keeping his chin down. He was pulling with his arms. He was making every stride laboriously, in an agony of willpower. But he was making it. He was running.

—Eddy Orcutt, "Wheelbarrow"

That is why athletes are important, why records are important. Because they demonstrate the scope of human possibility, which is unlimited. The inconceivable is conceived, and then it is accomplished.

—Brian Ganville, "The Olympian"

When he hears the gun, his muscles will automatically spring to action. He can almost feel the breeze that will flow smoothly over his face and arms and legs. His spikes will rhythmically splash cinder behind him and there will be cheering from the bleachers to his right.

—Louis Edwards, from the short story "Ten Seconds"

He felt good. Loose, with lots of juice in his flat-muscled body and an easy animal grace that brought the road back under him in long effortless strides.

—George Harmon Coxe, from the short story "See How They Run"

So, going downhill now, the enemy all around him, he experienced a sense of power, as though he were invisible, as though he were fleeter and stronger than anything that could seek to kill or hinder him. Sweat bathed him, he glistened as though oiled, and there was a slight froth at his lips. He moved with machinelike rhythm and his eyes - could they have been seen - might have seemed mad.

—Harry Sylvester, from the short story "Going to Run All Night"

The feel of that day was still in his limbs: he remembered the vague glow of promise, the sense of being released as he sped over the turf of roughly prepared track—effortless, as though his body had lightened, brought to a pitch of harmony by the simple miracle of the up-drawing sun.

—George Ewart Evans, from the short story "The Medal"

My eyes burned with sweat, and I squinted so tight I could hardly see anymore, and because they stung it was impossible to think. I was adjusting, though, lost in rhythm, like a mechanical animal caught on the rim of existence . . . it felt good and I was slipping deep in dreams.

—Walter McDonald, from the short story "The Track"

The runners would gather nervously at the starting line, taking care not to look each other in the eye.

—John L. Parker Jr., *Once a Runner*

Out of a silver heat mirage he ran. Two lanes of blacktop stretched straight and flat in front of him, straight and flat behind. August-tall corn walled in the road and its red-sand shoulders. A half mile away was a blue-dark wall of woods.

—James Tabor, from the short story "The Runner"

He ticked off six miles with reaching strides, his rhythm rolling on itself, like coasting downhill on oiled bearings.

—James Tabor, from the short story "The Runner"

[Running] transported him, taking his mind to another place, very deep within. Like prayer.

—Richard Christian Matheson, from the short story "Third Wind"

Running was the time he felt most alive. He knew that as surely as he'd ever known anything.

—Richard Christian Matheson, from the short story "Third Wind"

Look at me: a natural distance runner, wiry and muscular, trained down to gristle. We are the *infantry* of running. Your four-forty and eight-eighty men, these are your cavalry. The sprinters are your shock troops, your commandos.

—John L. Parker, Jr., *Once a Runner*

As he staggered, half-blind in the dim light, to the foot of the hill, he thought of the Athenian runner finishing the first Marathon and, as he collapsed, crying, "Rejoice, we conquer!" Nilson realized how much that image, those words had been with him, influencing him all his life. They heartened him now, sealed the sense of meaning in him.

—Harry Sylvester, "Going to Run All Night"

I waited for someone to speak, but all ran quietly, all alone. Now and then we would fall into step and there would be the thump thump thump of our running. Then the steps would syncopate and break rhythm and in the heavy depressing heat I would find myself having to concentrate to maintain stride.

—Walter McDonald, "The Track"

When the Literary Canon Goes Off

Wisely and slow. They stumble that run fast.

—Shakespeare, *Romeo and Juliet*

The long walk-run was still routine. He had fitted himself for the task; you did it daily and therefore could do it. The experience proved you could . . .If you stopped for a single day, much you had accomplished—at last got used to—you had to accomplish again.

—Bernard Malamud, *Dubin Lives*

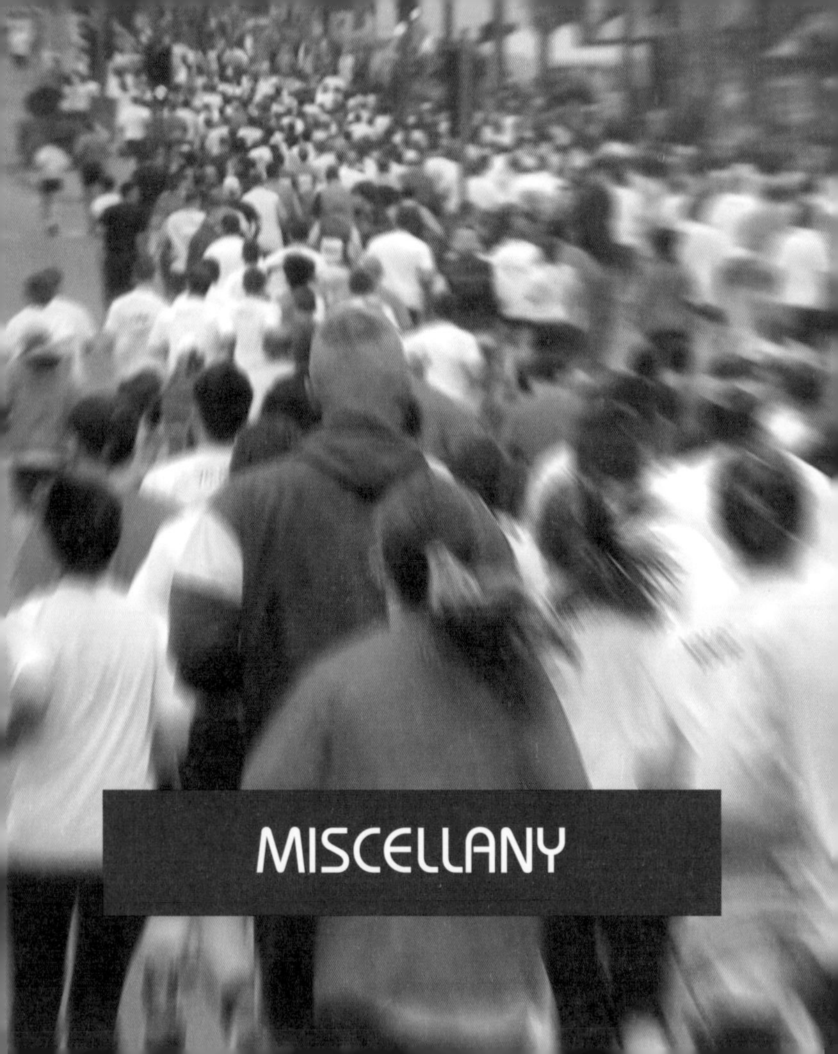
MISCELLANY

Miscellany

Miscellany is an ideal name for our final chapter. The term itself means "separate writings collected in one volume." Because the many writings and quotes about running included in this book have been culled from many different sources, it truly is a miscellany.

And if you are like me, I often read the last chapter first if it's a collection of quotes, essays or stories. (It's a habit I try to avoid at all costs when reading a novel or page-turning thriller.)

This chapter will provide you with a vivid snapshot (or kaleidoscopic look) of the broad diversity of wise, witty, and wonderful quotes pertaining to running that you will encounter elsewhere in this book. With that said, on your mark, get set . . ..

I've had a streak, and I'm into my prime years, but it ain't going to last forever.

—Bill Rodgers in 1979

Don't worry, everyone slows over time.

—Bill Rodgers

Running is a four-weather sport.

—Anonymous

The finishing line isn't given; it is earned.

—Anonymous

Run Now. Wine Later.

—Referring to a Thanksgiving race,
seen on *Runner's World's* online forum

Running a 12-minute mile still blows away sitting for 12 minutes on the couch.

—from *Runner's World's* online forum

The endurance athlete is the ultimate realist.

—Marty Liquori

Do or do not. There is no try.

—Yoda, from *Star Wars*

A man's errors are his portals of discovery.

— James Joyce

Our greatest glory is not never falling, but in rising every time we fall.

—Confucius

I pulled a hamstring during the New York City Marathon. An hour into the race, I jumped off the couch.

—David Letterman, on the New York City Marathon

Haile Gebrselassie is the best distance runner I have seen in the last quarter century, the most electrifying personality, and somewhat of an enigma, given his Ethiopian roots.

—Amby Burfoot

[I]t's only something normal for a sportsman to retire. You cannot control the whole world forever. People soon forget you because another champion comes along.

—Haile Gebrselassie

Every morning in Africa, an antelope wakes up. It knows it must outrun the fastest lion, or it will be killed. Every morning in Africa, a lion wakes up. It knows it must run faster than the slowest antelope, or it will starve. It doesn't matter whether you're the lion or an antelope – when the sun comes up, you'd better be running.

—African proverb

It's the road signs, "Beware of lions."

—Kip Lagat, Kenyan distance runner, during the Sydney Olympics, explaining why his country produces so many great runners

I was out training one black night when I heard a noise. I turned around and saw a leopard. I threw some stones at him and he went away, so I went on my way.

—Filbert Bayi, on running in his native Tanzania

For years, I've been in the habit of wearing running shoes everywhere and for every function. I even wear them with my tuxedo.

—Fred Lebow

[In 1971], America was more fascinated with competitive chess than with distance running.

—Edward McClelland

Lasse Viren, who I worked with in Finland, when he took his shirt off, he looked like a plucked chicken. There is no muscle there at all just ribs sticking out. He won four Olympic Gold Medals!

—Arthur Lydiard

If people saw you running in the street back then, they were likely to think you had stolen something.

—Arturo Barrios, former world-record holder in the 10,000 meters, on training in Mexico City, 1978

In the days of my victory and joy, I had faith enough to thank the Lord. Now, as well, I should not but accept my accident in grace.

—Abebe Bikila, a two-time Olympic Marathon champion, crippled in a car crash in 1969

Vision without action is a daydream. Action without vision is a nightmare.

—Japanese proverb

The nine inches right here; set it straight and you can beat anybody in the world.

—Sebastian Coe, pointing to his own head

Try to be better than yourself.

—William Faulkner

The thinking must be done first, before training begins.

—Peter Coe, father and coach to Sebastian Coe,
two-time Olympic gold-medalist in the 1,500 meters

The Empire is saved. Roar, Lion, Roar! There's been nothing to compare to this since the destruction of the Spanish Armada. England has the four-minute mile.

—Red Smith, sports columnist in the *International Herald Tribune*, May 8, 1954

When you get to the end of your rope, tie a knot and hang on.

—Theodore Roosevelt

There's nary an animal alive that can outrun a greased Scotsman.

—Groundskeeper Willy, from *The Simpsons*

For every finish-line tape a runner breaks—complete with the cheers of the crowd and the clicking of hundreds of cameras—there are the hours of hard and often lonely work that rarely gets talked about.

—Grete Waitz

To be a consistent winner means preparing not just one day, one month, or even one year—but for a lifetime.

—Bill Rodgers

I run 17 miles every morning. People ask me how I keep my teeth from chattering in the wintertime. I leave them in my locker.

—Walt Stack, starring in Nike's first "Just Do It" commercial (1988)

I didn't run a step from January of 1957 until August of 1963. I gained 40 pounds. I went up to about 200 from 160. In 1963 I felt the urge, the need to run. I started running 10 minutes out and back. I had no desire to run fast anymore. I had no desire to run 880s. I just wanted to run, and I'd run three or four days a week like that and I enjoyed it.

—Bruce Dern, regularly logged 100 miles per week in the 1960s, and later starred in the cult running film *On the Edge* (1986)

You want me to be your coach, you do what I say.

—Coach Elmo to Wes Holman (Bruce Dern), hoping for a running comeback at age 44, in *On the Edge*

Too short. Too short.

—Two Tarahumara, competing for Mexico, after finishing the 1928 Amsterdam Olympics marathon; race officials neglected telling them beforehand the course length, so they ran past the finish line until they were stopped

The Most Important Tip: Relax, it's just running. Of course it can be the most intoxicating, captivating, meaningful part of your life. But it's still just running. Nobody's making you do it, and you're not going to save the world doing it. So find what you enjoy about running, and then follow your bliss.

—Scott Douglas, *Little Red Book of Running*

Jane, stop this crazy thing!

—George Jetson, on treadmill

The single biggest change in middle-distance running, from the 1,500 meters to 10,000 meters, has been the track surface.

—Herb Elliott

Most mistakes in a race are made in the first two minutes, perhaps in the very first minute.

—Jack Daniels, exercise physiologist and coach

The only way to define your limits is by going beyond them.

—Arthur Clarke, author and futurist

I ran for myself, not Finland.

—Paavo Nurmi, aka "The Flying Finn," and world's best runner in the 1920s

Mind is everything: muscle—pieces of rubber. All that I am, I am because of my mind.

—Paavo Nurmi

Run into peace.

—Meister Eckhart, fourteenth-century philosopher

I run because long after my footprints fade away, maybe I will have inspired a few to reject the easy path, hit the trails, put one foot in front of the other, and come to the same conclusion I did: I run because it always takes me where I want to go.

—Dean Karnazes, celebrity ultrarunner

Now I am not running to please sponsors or to be the No.1 U.S. runner. Now I look at each step I get to take as a gift. I run because I love to run. I want to be able to run until I am 90 years old.

—Suzy Favor Hamilton, winner of nine NCAA individual titles

One cannot run away from his behind.

—African proverb

It was kind of an eye-opening thing, I started to feel old for the first time when I'm about two thirds of the way through a 5K and I'm going like, 'I'm working it. I'm doing good,' and look over and these two 8-year-olds passed me. They're like talking to each other, not even trying.

—Matt Damon, on a Thanksgiving Day fun run

Perhaps sometimes I was like a mad dog. It didn't matter about style or what it looked like to others; there were records to break.

—Emil Zatopek, who scored a distance-running gold-medal hat trick at 1952 Helsinki Olympics

[Zatopek] does everything wrong but win.

—Ohio State track coach Larry Snyder

Yesterday you said tomorrow.

—Nike quote

We told our guys to hold on for 30 minutes of agony for 12 months of glory.

—John McDonnell, Arkansas coach, after his runners won the 1993 NCAA Cross Country title

You can be an athlete. Athletes are very, very big in Coos Bay. You can study, try to be an intellectual, but there aren't many of those. Or you can go drag the Gut in your lowered Chevy with a switchblade in your pocket.

—Steve Prefontaine on his childhood in Coos Bay, Oregon

Pre{fontaine} was like Henry the Fifth. He didn't rule very long, but he left a big mark.

—Ken Kesey, author of *One Flew Over the Cuckoo's Nest*

Victory belongs to the most persevering.

—Napoleon Bonaparte

Things that hurt, instruct.

—Benjamin Franklin

Many of the things you can count, don't count. Many of the things you can´t count, really count.

—Albert Einstein

Success is counted sweetest by those who never succeed.

—Emily Dickinson

It is a sublime thing to suffer and be stronger.

—Henry Wadsworth Longfellow

[W]hen you actually race [famous runners], you don't want to hear about their being the stuff of legend. You want flesh and blood, preferably flesh covered with a slothful six or seven percent body fat and blood running a little low on hemoglobin. You want to see an arm action start to labor, a back stiffen. You want mortality, not legend.

—Kenny Moore

The coach would send us off on a long run—which then might be three miles—and Bill would be far more into it than me or the other guys. I'd take off and go to my girlfriend's house, but Bill would go run for an hour.

—Charlie Rodgers, Bill's brother, on their high-school cross country days

I introduced my wife to Billy, and afterwards she just couldn't believe he was the king of the roads. She thought he was just a mild-mannered schoolteacher from suburban Boston. And he was—until he laced on his shoes.

—Garry Bjorklund, Olympic runner and winner of numerous road races in the 1970s

Some people can't figure out what I'm doing. It's not a walk-hop, it's not a trot, it's running, or as close as I can get to running, and it's harder than doing it on two legs. It makes me mad when people call this a walk. If I was walking it wouldn't be anything."

—Terry Fox, cancer activist, who in 1980, ran for 143 days across Canada, covering 3,339 miles

You're really Frank Shorter, eh? What happened to you at Montreal?

—A Charleston, South Carolina cab driver upon learning he was driving Shorter, who won the Olympic gold in the marathon in 1972 and silver in 1976

In one of my early marathons I found myself unable to think of a single reason for continuing. Physically and mentally exhausted, I dropped out of the race. Now I won't enter a marathon unless I truly want to finish it. If during the race I can't remember why I wanted to run it, I tell myself, 'Maybe I can't remember now, but I know I had a good reason when I started.' I've finally learned how to fight back when my brain starts using tricky arguments.

—Jim Fixx, from *The Complete Book of Running*

Play not only keeps us young but also maintains our perspective about the relative seriousness of things. Running is play, for even if we try hard to do well at it, it is a relief from everyday cares.

—Jim Fixx

Clue in *New York Times* Crossword Puzzle on May 7, 2011: Best-selling jogging advocate

Answer: Jim Fixx

There were no spectators, only goats. I actually have a special feeling for goats, as we used to have them at home when I was growing up. But they don't make for a great cheering section.

—Fred Lebow on running the Aruba Marathon

Experienced runners learn to respect the changing needs of their bodies. That's the wisdom that comes with time, and—for good or bad—with age.

—Fred Lebow

In running, it doesn't matter whether you come in first, in the middle of the pack or last. You can say, 'I have finished.' There is a lot of satisfaction in that.

—Fred Lebow

Classical antiquity knew no such race as the marathon.

—Andrew Suozzo, author of *The Chicago Marathon*

For every runner who tours the world running marathons, there are thousands who run to hear the leaves and listen to the rain, and look to the day when it is suddenly as easy as a bird in flight.

—George Sheehan, M.D.

Methinks that the moment my legs began to move, my thoughts began to flow.

—Henry David Thoreau

Jogging is different from most popular physical fitness programs. Unlike weight lifting, isometric exercises and calisthenics with their emphasis on muscle building, jogging works to improve the heart, lungs, and circulatory system. Other body muscles are exercised as well, but the great benefit comes from improving the way the heart and lungs work. After all, when you are past 30, bulging biceps and pleasing pectorals may boost your ego, but your life and health depend upon how fit your heart and lungs are.

—Bill Bowerman and W.E. Harris, M.D., from *Jogging* (1967)

Walk breaks let you control the amount of fatigue on your legs and body.

—Jeff Galloway, from *Half-Marathon — You Can Do It*

Sharp runs so that the body may be emptied of moisture.

—Hippocrates

It is the athlete's job to learn to do the hard things easily.

—John Jerome, *The Sweet Spot in Time*

Run natural. Run free.

—Nick Pang, founder of MinimalistRunningShoes.org

On the better nights I dream of running fast again; light of feet and spirit and heart. It's way better than my dreams of sex and rock and roll.

—Scott Tinley, retired pro triathlete and two-time winner of the Hawaii Ironman

The thing about running is that when you can't do it any longer and are subjected to things like walking, spin classes and yoga, you miss it. Not the pain but everything else, which is everything.

—Scott Tinley

I did philosophy from miles five to eleven, trying to form one discriminating sentence about Socrates, Kant, Spinoza, Kierkegaard, whomever. When I came to the authors of *How to Be Your Own Best Friend*, I knew my mind was wandering and let go of systematizing.

—Max Apple, from the short story "Carbo-Loading"

Kids' shoes until recently have been marketed by the shoe companies to parents, educators, and health care professionals to prepare our kids for shoes they are marketing for adults to wear. The modern shoe industry and its marketing machine effectively convinces parents that when running, a child should wear miniature versions of traditional adult running shoes; almost all of which have elevated heels, extreme cushioning, and some form of motion-control technology. The next time you are in a park, watch a child run barefoot. Notice the relaxed movement and foot placement. They lean slightly forward and their legs fall out behind them. They do not strike hard on their heels. Then watch the child with the highly cushioned or supportive shoe. The difference is easy to see.

—Mark Cucuzzella, M.D.

It's rude to count people as you pass them. Out loud.

—Adidas ad

The whole issue is exactly that: getting enough calories. The first thing to worry about isn't so much what you eat, but how much you eat. You have to take the time to sit at the table and make sure your calorie count is high enough. And when you're a vegan, to increase your calories as you increase training you need more food. This isn't an elimination diet but an inclusion diet. If you go back 300 or 400 years, meat was reserved for special occasions, and those people were working hard. Remember, almost every long-distance runner turns into a vegan while they're racing, anyway — you can't digest fat or protein very well.

—Scott Jurek, elite ultrarunner and vegan

How many pairs of running shoes line your closet or clutter your doorstep? If you're typical of runners, you can count a half-dozen with mileage left in them. My current total is an even dozen.

—Joe Henderson

Q: Best advice from a runner?
A: It was from Rod Dixon. He said life is an elevator: you meet the same people on the way down as you do on the way up. So be careful how you treat people. Treat people (with respect), keep your word, and do the right thing because at some point you are not going to be good anymore and you never know, years down the road, when you might need the help of people.

—Steve Scott, one of U.S.'s greatest milers, in 2010 interview

Everything to me is the fit, the feel of the shoe. Do you feel biomechanically like you're moving barefoot? That's what you want. There is a trend now for simpler shoes. For 30 years I've thought they've had too many gimmicks on the running shoes. Various companies copying each other and trying to outdo each other and adding roll bars and computers on the shoes. It was unnecessary and made things more complicated than it should be.

—Bill Rodgers, in 2009 *New York Times* interview

There is reason for viewing with considerable apprehension the sudden popularity of the so-called Marathon race. It is only exceptional men who can safely undertake the running of twenty-six miles, and even for them the safety is comparative rather than absolute.

—*The New York Times*, February 24, 1909

When you run a marathon, you mean it. We're built for running. We dream of flying. For now, though, we're built to run.

—Benjamin Cheever, *Strides*

A long-sleeved shirt and shorts will always look better than a short-sleeved shirt with tights.

—Mark Remy, from *The Runner's Rule Book*

Running is meant to be enjoyed, not endured.

—Catherine McKiernan, retired Irish marathoner who won the London, Berlin, and Amsterdam Marathons, from foreword to *Chi Marathon*, by Danny Dreyer and Katherine Dreyer

You feel like if you're taking time off you didn't really earn it. But if you come out of a rested state, you perform better. After having trained so hard for so long and looking at other athletes, thinking, 'I trained 10 times harder than these guys and they're killing me in races,' you learn that more is not always better.

—Ryan Hall, whose 2:04.58 in the 2011 Boston Marathon was the fastest ever run by an American, in 2012 *Sports Illustrated* interview

I once ran thirty-one miles and after that there was nothing in the world I thought I couldn't do.

—Kathrine Switzer

ACKNOWLEDGEMENTS

In the process of putting together this brick of a book, I learned a lot about running and a little bit more about myself. I often found myself heading over to YouTube, where I'd watch video clips of great runners from the past—Bannister, Prefontaine, Zatopek, Wottle. Often times, my pulse would quicken as these runners headed down the home stretch. The head-bobbing Zatopek really did look as if he were being chased by zombies; yet the Czech Express set the modern standard of hard, intensive training.

Editing this book was part sprint, part marathon effort. Pacing was required, but toward the end, it was caffeine and insomnia that did the trick. I discovered that it's entirely possible to spend 18 hours in front of the computer, then make a strong cup of Sumatran-blend coffee and take a 30-minute run break around dawn, before getting back to the business of editing, researching and writing for another six hours...and then, with words dancing in my head but not making much sense, I knew that it was time to take a longer recess.

Acknowledgements

Friends and colleagues helped me with this book. My cohorts at the Natural Running Center—Mark Cucuzzella, M.D. and Nick Pang—offered their valuable insight and expertise. Nick's daughter, Claire, a high school cross-country and track-and-field athlete, did a stellar job assisting me with the organization of the quotes. Others I leaned on for their input: Steven Sashen, founder of Xero Shoes and truly the king of one-liners; Dr. Steve Gangemi aka "Sock Doc"; John Seery, who is also a night owl like myself; and Dr. Phil Maffetone for just being his usual wise self. Finally, Tony Lyons, publisher of Skyhorse Publishing, deserves credit for persuading me to do this book.

Bill Katovsky

THOSE QUOTED

Abrahams, Harold, British sprinter in Chariots of Fire

Allen, Mark, six-time Hawaii Ironman winner

Amar, Silvana, The Bedside Dream Dictionary

Apple, Max, author of the short story "Carbo-Loading"

Aristophanes, The Acharnians

Armstrong, Lance, seven-time Tour de France winner

Armstrong, Neil, astronaut

Averbuch, Gloria, author of health, fitness and running books

Ayres, Ed, co-founder of Running Times

Babington, John, longtime coach of the Wellesley College cross country and track team

Bacchylides, ancient Greek poet

Bannister, Roger, first person to break the four-minute mile

Barker, Molly, founder of Girls on the Run International

Barrios, Arturo, of Mexico and former world-record holder at 10,000 meters

Bayi, Filbert, runner from Tanzania

Beardsley, Dick, 1981 London Marathon champion and inducted into the National Distance Running Hall of Fame

Benoit-Samuelson, Joan, winner of the first-ever women's marathon at the 1984 Los Angeles Olympics

Benyo, Richard, editor of Marathon & Beyond and author of Timeless Running Wisdom

Berle, Milton, comic

Bikila, Abebe, a two-time Olympic Marathon champion, first-time barefoot in 1960 at Rome Olympics

Bingham, John, author of The Courage to Start

Bjorklund, Garry, Olympic runner and winner of numerous road races in the 1970s

Black, Andy, ultrarunner

Blaike, David, Canadian ultrarunner

Bloom, Marc, author ofThe Runner's Bible

Bolt, Usain, Jamaican gold medalist at the Beijing Olympics (100 meters, 200 meters, 4×100 meters relay team)

Bombeck, Erma, newspaper columnist

Bordin, Gelindo, winner of the 1988 Olympic Marathon in Seoul

Bowerman, Bill, co-founder of Nike, trained 24 NCAA champions and 16 sub-four-minute milers as coach at the University of Oregon

Bramble, Dr. Dennis, University of Utah biologist

Browning, Robert, "Pheidippides," "The Pied Piper of Hamelin"

Budd, Zola, former world-record holder in the women's 5,000 meters

Bunyan, John, Pilgrim's Progress (1678)

Burfoot, Amby, author of The Principles of Running, former editor-at-large at Runner's World, and winner of the 1968 Boston Marathon

Burleson, Dyrol, winner of the Compton Invitational Mile in 1964; Ryun, only 17, ran 3.59,0

Those Quoted

Carey, Drew, actor and host of The Price is Right
Carlin, George, comic
Carroll, Noel, top Irish middle-distance runner of the mid-1960s
Castella, Rob de, winner of 1983 World Marathon Championships, and won the 1981 Fukuoka Marathon in a world-record time of 2:08:18
Cather, Willa, author of Death Comes for the Archbishop
Cerutty, Percy, Australian running coach
Cheever, Ben, author of Strides: Running Through History With an Unlikely Athlete
Clarke, Arthur, author and futurist
Clarke, Ron, Australian distance runner and first man to break the 28-minute barrier in the 10,000 meters (27:39.4)
Coe, Peter, father and coach to Sebastian Coe, two-time Olympic gold-medalist in the 1,500 meters
Coe, Sebastian, of England, winner of the 1,500 meters in the 1980 and 1984 Olympics
Coghlan, Eamonn, of Ireland, and three-time Olympian and world-champion in the 5,000 meters
Combs, Sean "P. Diddy," music mogul
Conniff, Richard, Men's Health contributing writer
Cooper, Dr. Kenneth, author of 1968 best-seller Aerobics
Corbitt, Ted, known as the "father of long-distance running" and U.S. National Marathon Champion in 1954
Cordain, Loren, PhD, author of The Paleo Diet
Corneille, Pierre, author The Cid (1636)
Corre, Erwan Le, MovNat founder
Costill, David, professor of exercise science at Ball State University
Coubertin, Baron de, founder of the modern Olympics
Courtney, Tom, winner of the 800-meters final in the 1956 Melbourne Olympics
Coxe, George Harmon, author the short story "See How They Run"
Cucuzzella, Dr. Mark, owner of Two Rivers Treads, the nation's first minimalist shoe store, and winner of the 2011 Air Force Marathon
Culpepper, Alan, winner of the 2004 U.S. Olympic Marathon Trials

Damon, Matt, actor
Daniels, Jack, exercise physiologist and coach
Dante, poet
Davis, Dr. Irene, director of the Spaulding National Running Center at Harvard Medical School
Decker-Slaney, Mary, retired runner who set 36 U.S. middle-distance records
Deford, Frank, former Sports Illustrated writer
DeHaven, Rod, winner of U.S. 2000 Olympic Trials marathon (2:15:30)
Dekkers, Michelle, the barefoot South African runner who won the 1989 NCAA cross-country title for Indiana University
DeMar, Clarence, winner of seven Boston Marathons, beginning in 1910
Derderian, Tom, coach of the Greater Boston Track Club
Dern, Bruce, actor who starred in the cult running film. On the Edge (1986)
Dicharry, Jay, Director of the SPEED Performance Clinic and the Motion Analysis Lab Coordinator at the University of Virginia
Dixon, Rod, winner of the 1983 New York City Marathon
Doherty, Ken, 1928 American decathlon champion, author of the Track & Field

Omnibook, and long-time college track coach

Dolan, Liz, Nike's vice president for marketing

Douglas, Joe, founder of the Santa Monica Track Club whose athletes have won 27 Olympic medals and set 60 American records.

Douglas, Scott, author of Little Red Book of Running

Dreyer, Danny, author and co-founder of ChiRunning

Durden, Benji, ranked among the top ten U.S. marathoners for six consecutive years

Dwyer, Fred, Marty Liqouri's high school coach

Easton, Bill, legendary coach at Drake and University of Kansas, and whose teams won six NCCA titles

Eckhart, Meister, fourteenth-century philosopher

Edwards, Anthony, actor

Edwards, Louis, author ofthe short story "Ten Seconds"

Elliott, Jumbo, long-time Villanova track coach, on how runners should structure their lifestyle

Epictetus, ancient Greek philosopher

Epstein, Joseph, essayist

Escobar, Luis, seven-time finisher of the Western States 100

Evans, George Ewart, author of the short story "The Medal"

Ferrell, Will, actor

Finn, Adharanand, author of the book Running with the Kenyans

Fisher, Red, ultrarunner

Fixx, Jim, author of 1977 best-seller The Complete Book of Running

Flanagan, Shalane, winner of the 2012 U.S. Olympic Marathon Trials

Fleming, Tom, winner of the 1973 and 1975 New York City Marathon, and two time runner-up in the Boston Marathon

Fordyce, Bruce, nine-time winner of the Comrades Marathon in South Africa

Foster, Brendan, 3,000-meters world recorder in 1974

Fox, Terry, cancer activist, who in 1980, ran for 143 days across Canada, covering 3,339 miles

Foxx, Redd, comic

Galloway, Jeff, coach, author of Half-Marathon —You Can Do It

Gangemi, Dr. Steve, aka "Sock Doc," and 17-time Ironman finisher

Ganville, Brian, author of the short story "The Olympian"

Gareau, Jacqueline, 1980 Boston Marathon champion

Gebrselassie, Haile, Ethiopian running great and former world-record holder in the marathon

George, Walter, late nineteenth-century British runner whose world-record time in the mile (4:12) lasted for almost 30 years

Gibb, Roberta, first woman to "unofficially" run the Boston Marathon

Glover, Bob and Glover, Shelly-Lynn Florence, coauthosr of The Competitive Runner's Handbook

Gorman, Miki, two-time winner of Boston and New York City Marathons

Goucher, Adam, winner of 1999 U.S. Nationals 5,000 meters

Goucher, Kara, elite American long-distance runner who placed third at the 2012 U.S. Olympic marathon trials

Gray, Johnny, U.S. world-caliber 800-meters specialist who won a

bronze medal at the 1992 Barcelona Olympics
Gray, Thomas, "Ode on a Distant Prospect of Eton College"
Groundskeeper Willy, character in The Simpsons
Groves, Harry, Penn State coach
Guerrouj, Hicham El, of Morocco, world-record holder in the mile
Gump, Forrest, character in the movie Forrest Gump

Hall, Ryan, fastest Boston marathon (2011) time ever by an American, 2:04:58, finishing fourth
Hamilton, Suzy Favor, winner of nine NCAA individual titles
Hardy, Thomas, author of the novel Desperate Remedies
Heinrich, Bernd, Ph.D., author of Why We Run: A Natural History
Hemingway, Ernest, author and short-story writer
Henderson, Joe, writer, coach, and prolific author of running books
Higdon, Hal, prolific author of running books, with over 100 marathon finishes
Hill, Ron, elite British long-distance runner
Hollister, Geoff, University of Oregon runner and one of Nike's first employees
Homer, author of The Iliad
Homer, The Iliad
Hotz, Angie, aka "Barefoot Angie Bee" and run coach
Housman, A. E., author of To An Athlete Dying Young, from A Shropshire Lad (1896)
Huddle, Paul, multisport coach and former professional triathlete
Hussein, Ibraham, of Kenya and three-time winner of the Boston Marathon
Hutchins, Robert M., former President of the University of Chicago

Ibbotson, George Derek, mile world-record holder (3:57.2) in 1957
Ikangaa, Juma, of Tanzania, second-place Boston Marathon finisher three consecutive years and two-time winner of Tokyo Marathon

Jenner, Bruce, winner of the 1976 Olympic decathlon
Jennings, Lynn, one of the best female American distance runners of all time
Jensen, Stan, ultrarunner extraordinaire
Jerome, John, prolific fitness and travel author
Johnson, Ben, Canadian sprinter who forfeited gold medal in the 100 meters due to doping
Johnson, Brooks, Stanford University track and running coach
Johnson, Michael, winner of eight gold medals at the Worlds; and four Olympic gold medals (200 meters, 400 meters, and 4 x 400 meters relay)
Jones, Steve, former world-record holder in the marathon, and winner at the London, Chicago (twice), and New York City Marathons
Joyce, James, author of Portrait of the Artist as a Young Man
Joyner, Florence Griffith and Hanc, Jon, coauthors of Running for Dummies
Joyner-Kersey, Jackie, winner of three gold Olympic gold medals (heptathlon twice; long jump once).
Juantorena, Alberto, of Cuba, winner of 400 meters and 800 meters at the 1976 Olympics
Jurek, Scott, seven-time winner of Western States 100

Kardong, Don, author, journalist, coach, fourth-place finisher at the Montreal Olympic marathon
Karnazes, Dean, author of the bestselling Ultramarathon Man; and 11-time finisher (under 24 hours) of the Western States 100
Kastor, Deena, first American woman to run a marathon under 2:20
Katovsky, Bill, two-time Hawaii Ironman finisher, founder of Tri-Athlete, author, and editor of 1,001 Pearls of Running Wisdom
Keflezighi, Meg winner of the 2012 U.S. Olympic Marathon Trial
Keino, Martin, son of Kenyan running great Kipchoge Keino, and the 1994 NCAA cross country and 1995 NCAA 5,000-meters champion
Kelley, John A. "Old John," two-time winner of the Boston Marathon, which he finished 58 times
Kelley, John J. "Young John," Boston Marathon champion in 1957
Kennedy, Bob, U.S. 5,000-meters record holder and first non-African under 13 minutes
Kesey, Ken, author of One Flew Over the Cuckoo's Nest
Kipketer, Wilson Boit, Kenyan former world record-holder in the 3,000-meters steeplechase
Kipling, Rudyard, "If "
Kowalchik, Claire, author of The Complete Book of Running for Women
Kristiansen, Ingrid, of Norway, four-time winner of the London Marathon and two-time winner of the Boston Marathon
Krupicka, Anton, two-time winner of Leadville 100
Kuland, Lieutenant Colonel (Dr.) Dan, U.S. Air Force Chief of Health Promotion
Kuscsik, Nina, winner of Boston and New York City Marathons in 1972

Lagat, Kip, Kenyan distance runner
Lamppa, Ryan, a spokesman for Running USA, a nonprofit organization that tracks trends in running, on the rise of half-marathons
Lananna, Vin, Director of Track and Field for the University of Oregon and seven-time NCAA Coach of the Year
Landy, John, of Australia, and second runner to break four minutes in the mile
Larrieu, Francie, U.S. five-time Olympian
Lear, Chris, author of Running with the Buffaloes
Lebow, Fred, founder of New York City Marathon
Lebowitz, Fran, humorist and professional procrastinator
Lemons, Abe, college basketball coach
Letterman, David, TV talk-show host
Lewis, Carl, Olympic track and field star with nine gold medals
Lieberman, Daniel, Professor of Human Evolutionary Biology at Harvard University, aka "The Barefoot Professor"
Linenger, Jerry, NASA astronaut who spent 132 days aboard MIR
Liquori, Marty, top U.S. miler
Lister, Suzie, ultrarunner
Lloyd, J. William, writer of first treatise on running in 1890
Longfellow, Henry Wadsworth, author of "The Song of Hiawatha"
Lopes, Carlos, winner of the 1984 Olympic Marathon in Los Angeles, at age 37
Low, Dave, winner of Hawaii's Fittest CEO competition
Lydiard, Arthur, legendary New Zealand coach and father of Long Slow Distance (LSD) and "jogging"

Those Quoted

Mabe, Joan Nesbit, 1995 US Cross-Country National Champion and former Olympian
Macmillan, Don, Australian miler
Maffetone, Dr. Phil, author of The Big Book of Endurance Racing and Training
Magee, Barry, New Zealand, bronze medalist in the marathon at the 1960 Rome Olympics
Maitland, Sara, author of short story "The Loveliness of the Long-Distance Runner"
Malamud, Bernard, author of Dubin Lives
Marvell, Andrew, "To His Coy Mistress"
Masterkova, Svetlana, of Russia, gold-medalist in the 800 and 1,500 meters at the 1996 Olympics
Matheson, Richard Christian, author of short story "Third Wind"
McClelland, Edward, author and journalist
McClure, Walt, Steve Prefontaine's high school coach
McDonald, Walter, author of short story "The Track"
McDonnell, John, Arkansas track and field coach
McDougall, Christopher, author of Born to Run: A Hidden Tribe, Superathletes, and the Greatest Race the World Has Never Seen
McKiernan, Catherine, retired Irish marathoner who won the London, Berlin, and Amsterdam Marathons
McQueeney, Scott and Vivian, ultrarunning couple
Meyer, Greg, last American to win the Boston Marathon race (1983), in 2:09
Meyers, Rick, ultrarunner and owner of The Runner's Sole, a running specialty store in Chambersburg, Pennsylvania
Mills, Billy, winner of the 10,000 meters at the 1964 Tokyo Olympics
Mittleman, Stu, winner of the 1,000-Mile World Championship (11 days, 20 hours, 36 minutes) in 1986
Molina, Scott, one of the most dominant triathletes of the 1980s
Moller, Lorraine, four-time New Zealand Olympian
Montaigne, Michel de, Essays (1588)
Moore, Kenny, journalist and American fourth-place finisher in the 1972 Olympic Marathon
Morceli, Noureddine, of Algeria, and winner of the 1,500 meters at the 1988 Olympics
Morissette, Alanis, singer and actress
Morris, Desmond, best-selling British author of The Naked Ape
Moses, Edwin, two-time Olympic gold medalist in the 400-meters hurdles
Moss, Julie, retired professional triathlete
Mota, Rosa, three-time winner of Boston Marathon and Olympic gold-medalist in Seoul (1988)
Mull, Martin, comic
Murakami, Haruki, novelist and author of What I Talk About When I Talk About Running
Murray, Jim, Los Angeles Times sports columnist
Mussabini, Sam, British track coach featured in Chariots of Fire
Nelson, Kevin, author ofThe Runner's Book of Daily Inspiration
New York Road Runner's Club Complete Book of Running
Nieman, David, Ph.D., head of the Human Performance Laboratory, Appalachian State University
Nurmi, Paavo, aka "The Flying Finn," and world's best runner in the 1920s

O'Connor, Terry, (U.K.) Daily Mail journalist
O'Sullivan, Marcus, Irish three-time world-indoor champion in the 1,500 meters
Orcutt, Eddy, author of short story "Wheelbarrow"

Ortiz, Anita, winner of the 2008 Western States 100
Ovett, Steve, British gold medalist in the 800 meters at the 1980 Olympics, and former world-record holder in the 1,500 meters and mile (3:48)
Owens, Jesse, winner of four gold medals at the 1936 Berlin Olympics

Paige, Satchel, baseball pitcher
Pang, Nick, founder of MinimalistRunningShoes.org
Parker Jr., John L., author of Once a Runner
Pepys, Samuel, Samuel Pepys' Diary, July 30, 1663

Pindar, ancient Greek lyric poet
Pippig, Uta, of Germany, and the first woman to win the Boston Marathon three consecutive times (1994–1996)
Pisciotta, Jeff, Senior Researcher, Nike's Sports Research Lab
Pollan, Michael, author of In Defense of Food; and The Omnivore's Dilemma
Prefontaine, Ray, father of Steve Prefontaine
Prefontaine, Steve, U.S. top distance runner and track icon

Radcliffe, Paula, three-time winner of the London Marathon and two-time New York Marathon champion
Raines, Glen, aka "Barefoot Caveman"
Rang, Dr. Mercer, orthopedic surgeon and researcher in pediatric development
Ratelle, Alex, U.S. masters running great who clocked 18 flat in the 5K at the age of 64
Reinersten, Sarah, raced on the U.S. Disabled Track Team for 10 years, and first female leg amputee to finish the Hawaii Ironman
Remy, Mark, author of The Runner's Rule Book
Reynolds, Ryan, actor
Richardson, Charlotte Lettis, national caliber runner in the 1970s and winner of L'eggs Mini Marathon in Central Park in New York City
Rivers, Joan, ageless comic
Rob, Lil, Mexican-American music producer and rapper
Robillard, Jason, author of The Barefoot Running Book; editor and founder of The Barefoot Running University website
Robinson, Roger, author of Running in Literature; competitive runner for over 50 years
Rodgers, Bill, four-time winner of Boston and New York City Marathons
Rodgers, Charlie, Bill's brother
Romppanen, Eino, Finnish runner and sculptor
Rono, Henry, broke four world records in 81 days: 10,000 meters, 5,000 meters, 3,000 meters steeplechase, and the 3,000 meters
Rossi, Aldo, Italian poet
Royko, Mike, Chicago newsman
Rudd, Julie, U.S.miler Alan Webb"s wife
Rudisha, David Lekuta, Kenyan world-record holder in the 800 meters (1:41:09)
Rudner, Rita, comic
Rudolph, Wilma, winner of three gold medals in the 1960 Olympics (100 meters, 200 meters, and 4x100 meters relay)
Ryun, Jim, top U.S. miler in the 1960s who once held the world record

Salazar, Alberto, winner of Boston and three New York City Marathons
Sandrock, Michael, author of Running with the Legends
Santayana, George, philosopher